The Role of the Physical Therapist Assistant
Regulations and Responsibilities

SECOND EDITION

Holly M. Clynch PT, DPT, MA, GCS
Associate Professor/Program Director
Physical Therapist Assistant Program
St. Catherine University
Minneapolis, Minnesota

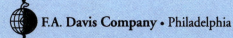 F.A. Davis Company • Philadelphia

F. A. Davis Company
1915 Arch Street
Philadelphia, PA 19103
www.fadavis.com

Copyright © 2017 by F. A. Davis Company

Printed in the United States of America

Last digit indicates print number: 10 9 8 7 6 5 4 3 2 1

Senior Acquisitions Editor: Melissa Duffield
Director of Content Development: George W. Lang
Developmental Editor: Rose Foltz
Design and Illustration Manager: Carolyn O'Brien

As new scientific information becomes available through basic and clinical research, recommended treatments and drug therapies undergo changes. The author(s) and publisher have done everything possible to make this book accurate, up to date, and in accord with accepted standards at the time of publication. The author(s), editors, and publisher are not responsible for errors or omissions or for consequences from application of the book, and make no warranty, expressed or implied, in regard to the contents of the book. Any practice described in this book should be applied by the reader in accordance with professional standards of care used in regard to the unique circumstances that may apply in each situation. The reader is advised always to check product information (package inserts) for changes and new information regarding dose and contraindications before administering any drug. Caution is especially urged when using new or infrequently ordered drugs.

Library of Congress Cataloging-in-Publication Data

Names: Clynch, Holly M., author.
Title: The role of the physical therapist assistant : regulations and
   responsibilities / Holly M. Clynch.
Description: Second edition. | Philadelphia : F.A. Davis Company, [2017] |
   Includes bibliographical references and index.
Identifiers: LCCN 2016038756 | ISBN 9780803658165
Subjects: | MESH: Physical Therapy Specialty—standards | Physical Therapist
   Assistants—standards | Practice Management—legislation & jurisprudence
Classification: LCC RM705 | NLM WB 460 | DDC 615.8/2023–dc23 LC record available at
https://lccn.loc.gov/2016038756

I dedicate this edition, as I did the first one, to my parents, Gil and Marcie Kehr, who raised me to believe I could accomplish anything I wanted; to my husband, Paul, whose encouragement and support have enabled me to accomplish so many things; and to my daughters, Blaire, Samantha and Michelle Hlavac, who will always be my greatest accomplishments.

This second edition is also dedicated to the memory of two special people who are no longer physically with us: my beloved brother, Pat Kehr and my dear friend and colleague Michael J. Baynes. I miss you both every day.

Acknowledgments

A book may be authored by an individual, but in reality, it cannot be produced without the support of so very many people. I must once again thank the following groups of people:

- My colleagues from the PTA and DPT faculty/staff at St. Catherine University. They are simply the best at what they do, and they motivate me every day to be the best that I can be, just to keep up with them. Much of the writing this time around was done while I was on sabbatical, and I especially want to thank Jessica Scholl and Susan Nelson for covering my duties during that time. Thanks also to the St. Kate's library staff, who were a tremendous help in updating my referencing software.
- All of the F.A. Davis people, especially Melissa Duffield, Senior Acquisitions Editor, and Rose Foltz, this edition's Developmental Editor. I continue to believe that Melissa knows more about physical therapy than anyone from outside the profession (and maybe more than some within it). One of the best perks of writing this book is the strong friendship I've developed with her—she's become the little sister I never had! And Rose not only made excellent suggestions for the new work I did this time around, but tightened up the existing material to make it even better than before. Thank you to both of you for putting up with all of my "life events" that interfered with my ability to stay on schedule.
- My mentors in the PT profession: Corinne Ellingham, Susan Sisola, and the late Marilyn Woods, each of whom believed in me enough to encourage me to take chances and push myself in new directions. A special word of gratitude goes to Susan, from whom I took over the "Introduction to Physical Therapy/Role of the PTA" course at St. Kate's. Although I have tweaked it in the years since then, much of the course's (and, therefore, this textbook's) content began as a product that she put together.
- My best-ever friend Annie, who is always there for me, believing in me 100% of the time. Thank you for understanding when I had to cancel plans with you because I was behind schedule on this!
- My wonderful family. In addition to my parents, husband, and daughters who were singled out in the dedication, I must also thank my siblings, sibs-in-law and their families. I know they don't really understand why and what I do in the world of PT or academia, but they've never questioned whether or not I had the ability to do it. Thanks especially to Sheila and John for once again providing a place for me to get away and write in isolation. This time they set up an office for me in their lovely Mexican home … truly the best place to spend a winter sabbatical!
- And, last but not least, my incredible former and current students at St. Catherine University. Their efforts and their sacrifices never cease to amaze me. They motivate me to be a better instructor, and I am honored to be part of their educational process.

I am blessed to have such a wonderful network of support—once again, you all had a piece in this!

Preface

Writing this book has been one of the highlights of my career, and I am honored to have been given the opportunity to update it for a second edition. This book is as much about the "relationships, relevance, and role modeling" required in the PT/PTA relationship as it is about the "rules, regulations and responsibilities" that one might expect from the title of the book. I wrote this book because I struggled to find a textbook that addressed all of these "Rs" to my satisfaction. Changes in health care and the evolution of the physical therapy profession have led to confusion, misinterpretation and disagreement on what the PT/PTA relationship should look like. It is obvious to me that both PTs and PTAs need to have a greater, more uniform understanding on the parameters of the PTA's role in the clinic, and to have more clear expectations regarding the preferred PT/PTA relationship. This interaction is at the core of the PTA's work – the PTA cannot exist without it!

What's New in the Second Edition? What's the Same?

In the past five years, there have been many changes in the physical therapy world...a new, outwardly focused vision statement, changes in APTA positions and third-party payment rules, and an increased focus on the physical therapist's role as a primary care provider. Specific to the PTA, the APTA House of Delegates has debated the use of the PTA versus other support personnel, has discussed the PTA's educational needs at entry-level and beyond, and has created a mechanism for chapters and sections to grant PTAs a full voice in component voting. It's my personal belief that there has never been a better time to be a physical therapist assistant, and I hope that the changes made in the second edition reflect the more positive environment for PTAs within the APTA.

In addition to the general editing and updating that occurred in every chapter, more significant additions/revisions, based on reviewer feedback, include the following:

- Due to popular demand, a new chapter was added, Chapter 11, "Payment for Physical Therapist Services." This chapter was one that I resisted writing in the first edition out of concern that it would soon contain out-of-date information, due to the ever-changing payment environment. However, my readers convinced me that students needed some type of introduction to the health care systems impacting the delivery of physical therapy prior to going out on clinical experiences. Depending on when that occurs in a particular program, it might be a chapter that is deferred until later in the curriculum.

- Chapter 9, "The Physical Therapist Assistant and the American Physical Therapy Association," was moved from its previous location as Chapter 3, based on instructor feedback that they weren't using it early in the curriculum. It has been updated to include recent PTA-related decisions by the House of Delegates and the Board of Directors. These outcomes helped with my deliberate effort to make the tone of this chapter more positive than in the previous edition.
- "Laws Impacting Physical Therapist Practice" has also been moved to later in the book (now Chapter 10), for the same reasons, and now includes information about the Americans with Disabilities Act
- Chapter 2, "Physical Therapist Practice Settings," includes updated information related to the new edition of the *Guide to Physical Therapist Practice* and more detailed content/questions related to the ICF model of patient categorization. The principles of interprofessional education and discussion questions about the other providers with whom the PTA might interact are also included in this chapter.
- Expanded information about electronic medical records and a discussion about point-of-service documentation are addressed in the "Introduction to Documentation" chapter (now Chapter 8).

As in the first edition, the biggest challenge continues to be finding the best way to present material that is sometimes thought of as less "exciting" (yet no less important) than other content in a physical therapy program. I've received lots of positive feedback on the Reflection Bullets found throughout the chapters, as well as on the Review and Application sections at each chapter's end. Some of them have been edited, usually because my own students were having trouble interpreting what was being asked in the question! Others have been changed to reflect revisions in the content or to better address the key concepts in the chapter. I've also tried to avoid questions that ask students to go to a particular website, as I've learned that web addresses frequently become obsolete even faster than the general content in the book. Especially in the later chapters, I've tried to incorporate content and questions which might be more appropriate for use later in the curriculum, after students have performed clinical experiences. I hope that the bullets and questions in the book (whether used during individual reading, with a partner, or as part of class discussions or assignments) serve as reminders to stop and think about why this material is being presented and how it impacts you, your colleagues and the patients with whom you will interact.

Unique Features of This Book

As in the first edition of the book, there were a few deliberate decisions that were made in choosing how to present the material in this textbook. Part of the challenge of developing a book like this is that the state statutes, especially in regard to the PTA, are so variable. Therefore, there are few state-specific examples of regulations included within the text. It is assumed that the reader understands, first and foremost, that state laws must be followed in the provision of physical therapy services. Having said that, it is also clear, in reviewing those statutes, that many are silent as to the specifics of what the PTA can and cannot perform, or how the PTA should be supervised. The book places a heavy emphasis on current APTA policies and positions, and that is deliberate. Especially when practice acts are silent, I believe that the APTA is the best resource for defining and refining the scope of work for the PTA and the PT/PTA relationship. Again, the reader may not always agree with current policies or policy-makers. If not, I challenge you to become more involved in association work.

Another issue in writing this book was in deciding how to refer to those individuals who benefit from physical therapy services. As explained in Chapter 2, the APTA's *Guide to Physical Therapist Practice* recommends the use of the term "patient/client" when referring generically to the population that utilizes physical therapy, and is the term used in the Association documents that you will see highlighted and referenced throughout this textbook. However, as this book's original content was written and reviewed, using the term "patient/client" often seemed awkward or interfered with the flow of the material being presented. Therefore, with no disrespect intended to the Guide's developers, I have chosen to use the term "patient" in this textbook as the primary term defining those people for whom PTs and PTAs provide services. It should be understood by the reader that, in this book, the term "patient" may include other individuals beyond those who are seen in the traditional medical context of physical therapy.

In the second edition, even more than the first, I wanted to avoid using gender-specific pronouns, but the flow of the material often requires use of a specific pronoun. Therefore, I have continued to use only one gender-specific pronoun, he or she, in each chapter. Because of the resequencing of some chapters, sometimes there are two chapters in a row that use the same pronoun. However, the total number of chapters are evenly split. It is hoped that this formatting choice continues to be as inclusive as possible without sacrificing clarity.

Using This Book—In School and Beyond

Successfully creating the preferred PT/PTA relationship starts with DPT and PTA academic programs but must be carried out in the clinic. It was my intent to write this text in such a way that (hopefully) it can be used throughout the time during which one is a student and also during one's career as a PTA or PT. We all know that it is impossible to retain every fact and concept to which we are exposed during school. I have always maintained that part of the role of an academic program is not to ensure that students "know everything" when they leave, but to teach them where and how to find information (knowledge that they either have "forgotten" or never learned) as they prepare for, begin, and progress in their careers. I hope that this textbook serves both of those purposes. It can function as a guide for ensuring a thorough knowledge base about the role of the PTA and about appropriate day-to-day interaction between PTs and PTAs – something for which both PTs and PTAs are responsible – and can also serve as a resource for those who need to find more in-depth information about a particular subject. I have found that many practicing PTs who didn't receive much education about the role of the PTA are especially appreciative of having the information provided here. For those of you who are (or will be) PTAs, you might consider sharing this textbook with coworkers who are less familiar with your education, how PTAs should perform in the clinic and/or how PTs should appropriately provide supervision for them.

As is appropriate for an introductory textbook, many of the chapters present basic information regarding subjects on which entire textbooks have been written. If and when you need more information on one of these subjects, use the citations within each chapter to lead you to sources which address it in greater depth (they have all been updated to include newest editions of books and more current articles.) I have attempted to compile entry-level "need to know" information on a breadth of subjects, but many of my brilliant colleagues have a greater depth of knowledge to share about them—refer to their materials, and use their expertise to increase yours.

One cannot help but notice the frequent references in this book to APTA policies, positions, and activities. In performing the extensive research that goes along with writing and rewriting a book, I've continued to be impressed with how much our association does for our profession and for everyone who is part of it – PTs, PTAs, students and, most importantly, our patients. I hope that this textbook will help each reader develop a greater awareness of (and gratitude for) all that the APTA does, and why every PT and PTA needs to be involved with the APTA at some level. As previously stated, the profession of physical therapy and the work of the APTA are constantly evolving, and the information included here is only as current as the day it was written. The best way to stay up to date on what is happening in the profession of physical therapy is to be an APTA member. The benefits far outweigh the expense, and hopefully this book will help readers to recognize this.

Thank you once again for giving me the opportunity to share my vision, based on the evidence of current laws, APTA positions, and research, combined with my personal clinical and teaching experience, for what the PT/PTA relationship should look like. Sharing that vision with you, the reader, is what this book is all about. You may not agree with the components of my vision, but it is my hope that any disagreement will lead to further research and debate, serving to further unify our profession's utilization of the PTA.

Reviewers

Frank Bates, PT, DPT, MBA
Krannert School of Physical Therapy, College of
    Health Sciences
University of Indianapolis
Indianapolis, Indiana

Nijah Chinn-Gonsalves, PT, DHS
Physical Therapist Assistant
ECPI University
Richmond, Virginia

Matthew M. Connell, PTA
Physical Therapist Assistant
State College of Florida
Bradenton, Florida

Rebecca Crocker, PT, DPT
Physical Therapist Assistant Program
Ozarks Technical Community College
Springfield, Missouri

Anna Lapinski, DPT
Physical Therapist Assistant
SOLEX College
Chicago, Illinois

Heather MacKrell, PT, PhD
Health Sciences
Calhoun Community College
Decatur, Alabama

Danette Neikirk, MPT
Physical Therapy
Cape Girardeau CTC
Cape Girardeau, Missouri

Diana Ploeger, PT, M Ed
Physical Therapist Assistant
Salt Lake Community College
West Jordan, Utah

Elisa Marie Zuber, PT, PhD
Physical Therapist Assistant Program
South University, High Point
High Point, North Carolina

Contents

The History of Physical Therapy and the Physical Therapist Assistant

CHAPTER OBJECTIVES

After reading this chapter, the reader will be able to:

- Identify key events in the early development of the physical therapy profession.
- Discuss the factors that led to the creation of the physical therapist assistant (TA) position.
- Describe the initial concerns and issues related to PTA task delegation and skill performance.
- Identify historical and current trends in demands for PTA services and PTA educational program enrollment.
- Compare and contrast the use of the term "professional" versus "professionalism" in regard to the PTA.
- Discuss the profession's focus for the future as outlined in the vision statement of the American Physical Therapy Association (APTA).

KEY TERMS AND CONCEPTS

- Rehabilitation
- Reconstruction aides
- Physical Therapist Assistant
- Professionalism in Physical Therapy: Core Values
- Values-Based Behaviors for the Physical Therapist Assistant
- Autonomous practice
- Direct access
- APTA Vision Statement for Physical Therapy
- Movement System

F*rancine is a high school senior interested in working in a health-care field. When she sprains her ankle during a softball game, her physician says she will need to go to physical therapy. "What's that?" Francine wonders. At the local outpatient clinic, she is seen by Sofia, a physical therapist (PT), who tells Francine what physical therapy is and how the profession began. Francine becomes very interested. However, she is discouraged to find out that she needs to go to school*

(vignette continues on page 2)

for 6 to 7 years to become a PT. "You could consider becoming a PTA," Sofia tells her. Francine asks, "What is a PTA? Is that the same as a PT aide? How long do they have to go to school? How is that different from being a PT?"

QUESTIONS TO CONSIDER

How did the profession of physical therapy begin? What needs led to the development of the PTA position? What educational degree is awarded to a PTA?

This chapter reviews the history of the physical therapy profession and the factors that led to the development of the PTA. It addresses the current status of PTA education and employment and how these may change based on future goals and trends within the profession. It also begins to identify concepts and positions that are used by the APTA to differentiate the role of the PTA from that of the PT, a theme that continues throughout this textbook.

The Beginnings of Physical Therapy

People have always used touch, water, and heat to soothe and comfort.[1] It was from these interventions that the profession of physical therapy has developed. Over the years, the application of these and many other techniques has been researched, applied, and refined, leading to what is now recognized as physical therapy practice.

The profession of physical therapy developed in part as a result of two major events: the polio epidemic of the early 1900s and World War I. Patients (often children) who contracted polio sustained temporary or permanent paralysis and muscle atrophy because of the disease process and the prolonged bedrest associated with it. Meanwhile, because of advances in medical treatment, soldiers injured in World War I survived their injuries at a much higher rate than did soldiers in previous wars, but they were having difficulty returning to duty or civilian life.[2] Both groups of patients required **rehabilitation,** the process of treatment and education to improve their functional skills and maximize their level of independence,[3] to facilitate their return to previous levels of physical performance. The need for rehabilitation services therefore led to an increased need for those with formal training to provide those services.

Mary McMillan, born in the United States but trained in England, is widely considered the first PT. In 1918, she was appointed to lead a group of women being trained as **reconstruction aides,** as the early PTs were then called. These women learned how to use hydrotherapy (therapeutic use of water), exercise, and massage to promote healing and strengthening. After training, they were sent to Europe to "reconstruct" the soldiers injured in the war (Fig. 1-1).[4] By the war's end, physiotherapists, as they came to be known, continued to work with children with

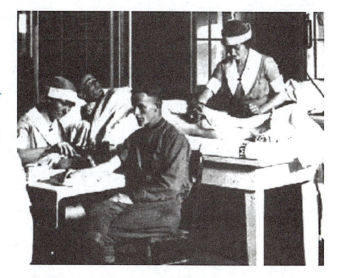

Figure 1-1. Early PTs Performing Exercises With Soldiers at Fort Sam Houston, Texas. (Reprinted with permission of the American Physical Therapy Association. This material is copyrighted, and any further reproduction or distribution requires written permission from APTA.)

polio and expanded their training to include more in-depth study in the use of physical agents (such as heat, cold, light, and electricity) that were used to cause desired physiological changes.[3] The onset of World War II and its aftermath, along with additional polio outbreaks, led to a renewed need for PTs (as they began to be called in the United States in the 1940s) to serve military personnel as well as the general public. Physical therapy expanded its service delivery to others besides soldiers and children, providing those services in a variety of settings, including nursing homes, hospitals, and rehabilitation centers, and the need for skilled providers continued to grow.[2]

In the 1940s, the profession began to discuss the need for formally trained assistants.[5] However, in the 1960s, with a limited number of PTs available and the training time having increased to a minimum of that required for a bachelor's degree,[6] the profession began a more thorough investigation into alternative mechanisms for cost-effective care delivery. In her 1965 Mary McMillan Lecture, former APTA president Catherine Worthingham stated that the training of assistants needed to "be faced quickly and in a manner that is in the best interests of the patient and our developing profession."[7] The perceived need for more providers grew even stronger in 1967, when the newly developed Medicare system added physical therapy as a reimbursable skilled service.[2]

Development of the PTA

As the need for some type of support personnel became apparent, there was a desire to have this new support position educated in a uniform fashion. Therefore, in 1967, the APTA House of Delegates adopted the policy "Training and Utilization of the Physical Therapy Assistant," which outlined the anticipated role, function, and educational expectations.[8] Eventually, the title **"physical therapist assistant"** was deliberately chosen over "physical therapy assistant" to reflect that the role was to directly assist the PT in the delivery of services.[4] APTA then worked with the accrediting body now known as the Commission on Accreditation for Physical Therapy Education (CAPTE) to develop uniform educational standards for the PTA, with a degree to be awarded at the associate (2-year) level. In 1967, Miami Dade Community College (now Miami Dade College) and St. Mary's Junior College (now St. Catherine University) admitted and began educating students for the role of the PTA. In 1969, these first PTAs graduated and began working in the clinic alongside PTs.[5]

From the beginning, despite PTAs' uniform education and the APTA's attempt to standardize their role, there was debate over how the services of the PTA should be utilized. There was a deliberate emphasis in the new educational programs to train PTAs to do more than just perform physical therapy services. From the beginning, despite uniform educational standards and the APTA's attempt to standardize the PTA's role, PTs debated how to utilize the services provided by PTAs. The new educational programs to train PTAs deliberately emphasized doing more than performing physical therapy skills. These students became educated in the theories and principles of physical therapy, enabling them to perform as technicians without the constant direct oversight of the PT.[4] Some PTs even suggested that because of the technical emphasis of their training, PTAs might have a higher skill set in some areas than did the PT.[8] Many PTs feared that the PTA would "take over" the day-to-day interaction with the patient, which was a favorite part of the PT's role. Others worried that the PTA would be given too much responsibility for patient care.

In 1971, Dr. Nancy Watts published a landmark article that described the factors that the PT should consider when delegating tasks to a PTA. Dr. Watts advocated against only using a "checklist" of skills permissible for the PTA. She encouraged the supervising PT to use a process of decision-making and discretion in delegating tasks, considering the skills and abilities of each PTA relative to several factors, including the following:

- The complexity of the task, the amount of "decision-making" versus "doing" involved with that task, and the risks involved (including the predictability of the situation and the clarity of the choices to be made)
- The criticality/stability of the patient and severity of the consequences if an error in task performance were to be made
- The purpose of the task in relation to treating the patient's problem versus contributing to the patient's sense of well-being and satisfaction with the overall provision of services
- The experience, areas of specialization, and unique body of knowledge possessed by both the PT and the PTA[9]

Watts's article is still used by both PT and PTA educators as a method of explaining the complexity of the decision-making that should be involved in task delegation.

FOR REFLECTION

FOR REFLECTION

- If PTAs are being educated in a uniform manner, why do PTs need to take all these factors into consideration when deciding what to delegate? Shouldn't all PTAs be able to perform all tasks in which they have been educated?

Demand for PTA Services

As the profession of physical therapy has grown, so has the demand for the PTA. In the 1980s and 1990s, the number of PTA programs throughout the country increased rapidly in response to a need for increased physical therapy services in schools, skilled nursing facilities, and other health-care settings. Despite the consistency of CAPTE educational standards, as the number of PTA programs grew, so did the variations in graduate performance and skill sets. The variation in the abilities of these new graduates (based in part on some early PTA educators having limited experience in teaching and with the role of the PTA), combined with the advanced clinical experience of the original PTA graduates, led to even greater confusion and debate about the appropriate role and utilization of the PTA.[5] Uncertainty and disagreement on this subject continue and are discussed later in this chapter.

In the mid- to late 1990s, the job market in physical therapy was beginning to show signs of saturation as more PTs and PTAs graduated each year from an increasing number of educational programs. This number reached a tipping point when, in 2000, reimbursement changes brought about by implementation of the federal government's 1997 Balanced Budget Act (BBA) resulted in nationwide staffing changes.[6] Many PTs and PTAs lost their positions owing to decreased facility revenue from physical therapy and other health-care services. Because of the saturated job market, many PTA programs saw their enrollment significantly reduced, and other programs were forced to close or go to a temporary "inactive" status. In 2001, the overall number of PTA programs dropped for the first time since the beginning of PTA education.[10] However, modifications of those initial BBA reimbursement regulations coupled with an overall aging population and the increasing prevalence of chronic health conditions later resulted in a rebound in the need for skilled services. In the second decade of the 21st century, the number of new educational programs is once again on the rise, with many more PTA than PT programs currently in development.[10] There are many possible reasons for the prevalence of new PTA programs, all of which may make a PTA program appear to be a more appealing route for entering the physical therapy profession. These reasons include the following:

- The difference in costs and duration of an associate degree program versus graduate-level education
- The smaller number of educational prerequisites required for entering a PTA program
- The differences in academic focus, especially in light of the fact that the entry-level PT degree is now primarily awarded at the doctoral level
- The perceived differences in the daily time commitments that might be required of students in each program

Currently, there is discussion within the profession about whether the associate degree level of education sufficiently prepares the PTA for today's expectations for entry-level clinical performance. Although the APTA acknowledges changes in practice that support the need for additional PTA education, it continues to support the associate degree as the required entry-level degree.[11] However, a number of PTA programs are currently investigating the development of bachelor's degree programs, and it is possible that in the future the required entry-level PTA degree may change. This issue is addressed in greater detail in Chapter 9.

FOR REFLECTION

- Return to the scenario in the beginning of this chapter. Imagine that Francine asks you why you have chosen this career path. In your own words, explain why you chose your particular educational program.

Current Utilization of the PTA

As mentioned, the debate continues regarding how PTAs should be utilized. Today's clinical environment generally requires a higher level of decision-making and critical thinking than that which existed at the time the PTA position was created.[12] Variations in utilizations may occur based on state regulatory requirements or because of an individual facility's PT/PTA utilization policy or philosophy (for example, a facility might expect a PT to see the patient for some part of every clinic visit). Differences in utilization also may occur based on the supervising PT's familiarity with the role of the PTA and the PTA's educational skill set, the PT's comfort level in directing and providing supervision for the PTA, and the PTA's ability to take responsibility. All these issues, along with their impact on service delivery and patient care, are addressed in subsequent chapters. Chapter 3 specifically explores the preferred PT/PTA relationship and the factors that can determine the success of the team.

The APTA has developed and refined a number of core documents, standards, and positions that define the role and utilization of the PTA. The position statement "Distinction Between the Physical Therapist and Physical Therapist Assistant in Physical Therapy"[13] addresses terms used to differentiate the PT from the PTA. This specific position also states that "the practice of physical therapy is conducted by the physical therapist,"[13] which at first glance may be interpreted as not being inclusive of the PTA. However, it is important to note that other APTA positions define "physical therapist practice" as including "utilization of physical therapist assistants who assist with selected components of intervention."[14]

Distinction Between the Physical Therapist and the Physical Therapist Assistant in Physical Therapy (HOD P06-01-18-19)

The American Physical Therapy Association (APTA) is committed to promoting the physical therapist as the professional practitioner of physical therapy and promoting the physical therapist assistant as the only individual who assists the physical therapist in the provision of selected physical therapy interventions. APTA is further

Distinction Between the Physical Therapist and the Physical Therapist Assistant in Physical Therapy (HOD P06-01-18-19) (continued)

committed to incorporating this concept into all Association policies, positions, and program activities, wherever applicable.

Professional: The term "professional," when used in reference to physical therapy services, denotes the physical therapist.

Physical Therapist Assistant: The physical therapist assistant is an educated individual who works under the direction and supervision of a physical therapist. The physical therapist assistant is the only individual who assists the physical therapist in accordance with APTA's policies and positions in the delivery of selected physical therapy interventions. The physical therapist assistant is a graduate of a physical therapist assistant education program accredited by the Commission on Accreditation in Physical Therapy Education.

Practice: The practice of physical therapy is conducted by the physical therapist.

Another confusing element of this position relates to its definition of the term "professional." According to this position, the term refers only to the PT and therefore should not be used to describe a PTA. PTAs should understand that the rationale for that distinction relates to the historical definition of a "profession"; one facet of this definition states that professionals have autonomy in decision-making.[15] Because by design PTAs must perform their duties under the direction and supervision of a PT, they do not have the same level of autonomy as do PTs. However, some physical therapy clinicians argue that the PTA is:

- Expected to make independent decisions regarding the patient's status and response during the course of a given intervention, and
- Allowed to modify the interventions independently (within the plan of care) when in the best interests of the patient.

Those clinicians believe, therefore, that the PTA does have some autonomy and should be considered one specific type of professional in physical therapy.[15] Others maintain that because some jurisdictions and third-party payers limit the physical therapist's autonomy, using the traditional criteria to determine a professional also excludes the PT. In fact, in many arenas physical therapy continues to be labeled as an "allied health profession" along with many other fields with less training and less autonomy. The APTA encourages activity that eliminates this terminology from statutes, health-care policy documents, and other venues.[16]

Pellegrino argues that the definition of "profession" and "professional" in health care has less to do with the traditional criteria or the credentials one has, and more to do with the position of power that that health-care providers hold over their patients/clients, and the unique interpersonal relationship that they establish with their patients

Table 1-1 Traditional vs. Contemporary Criteria for Determining a Professional (as proposed by Pellegrino)[17]

Traditional	Contemporary
Service to clients	Provider works with patients in need of help
Specialized education	Patient needs are personal with high impact on life
Representative organization	Patients become vulnerable, give up confidentiality
Autonomy of judgment	Provider offers knowledge, promise of help
Lifetime commitment	Patient "forced" to place trust in provider

(see Table 1-1).[17] This view of professional behavior, inclusive of the PTA, is reinforced throughout this text, especially in Chapter 6, which addresses the responsibilities of the PTA in developing strong interpersonal relationships with patients/clients.

FOR REFLECTION

- Compare and contrast the attributes and how they are defined in each document. How do the variations within each document reflect the differing roles of the PT and PTA? Are there any differences or similarities that surprise you?

The PTA role has many characteristics that fall under the category of "professionalism" as identified by the APTA. One of its core documents, **"Professionalism in Physical Therapy: Core Values,"**[18] although not developed for the PTA, is used by many PTA educational programs to identify those traits that PTA graduates are expected to demonstrate. A PTA-specific document, **"Values-Based Behaviors for the Physical Therapist Assistant,"** includes many of the same attributes, though not always defined in the same way because of the differences in the roles of the PT and PTA.[19] Both documents provide examples of how these behaviors might be demonstrated in the clinical setting, and have accompanying self-assessments tools that allow clinicians to identify areas in need of further development. These assessments can be found on the APTA website.

Professionalism in Physical Therapy: Core Values (BOD P05-04-02-03)

Accountability

Accountability is active acceptance of the responsibility for the diverse roles, obligations, and actions of the physical therapist including self-regulation and other

Professionalism in Physical Therapy: Core Values (BOD P05-04-02-03) (continued)

behaviors that positively influence patient/client outcomes, the profession, and the health needs of society.

Altruism

Altruism is the primary regard for or devotion to the interest of patients/clients, thus assuming the fiduciary responsibility of placing the needs of the patient/client ahead of the physical therapist's self-interest.

Compassion/Caring

Compassion is the desire to identify with or sense something of another's experience; a precursor of caring. Caring is the concern, empathy, and consideration for the needs and values of others.

Excellence

Excellence is physical therapy practice that consistently uses current knowledge and theory while understanding personal limits, integrates judgment and the patient/client perspective, embraces advancement, challenges mediocrity, and works toward development of new knowledge.

Integrity

Integrity is steadfast adherence to high ethical principles or professional standards; truthfulness, fairness, doing what you say you will do, and "speaking forth" about why you do what you do.

Professional Duty

Professional duty is the commitment to meeting one's obligations to provide effective physical therapy services to patients/clients, to serve the profession, and to positively influence the health of society.

Social Responsibility

Social responsibility is the promotion of a mutual trust between the profession and the larger public that necessitates responding to societal needs for health and wellness.

Values-Based Behaviors for the Physical Therapist Assistant

Altruism

Altruism is the primary regard for or devotion to the interests of the patient/client, assuming responsibility of placing the needs of the patient/client ahead of the PTA's self interest.

(box continues on page 10)

Values-Based Behaviors for the Physical Therapist Assistant (continued)

Caring and Compassion
Compassion is the desire to identify with or sense something of another's experiences; a precursor of caring. Caring is the concern, empathy, and consideration for the needs and values of others.

Continuing Competence
Continuing competence is the lifelong process of maintaining and documenting competence through ongoing self-assessment, development, and implementation of a personal learning plan, and subsequent reassessment.

Duty
Duty is the commitment to meeting one's obligations to provide effective physical therapy services to individual patients/clients, to serve the profession, and to positively influence the health of society.

Integrity
Integrity is the steadfast adherence to high ethical principles or standards; truthfulness, fairness, doing what you say you will do, and "speaking forth" about why you do what you do.

PT/PTA Collaboration
The PT/PTA team works together, within each partner's respective role, to achieve optimal patient/client care and to enhance the overall delivery of physical therapy services.

Responsibility
Responsibility is the active acceptance of the roles, obligations, and actions of the PTA, including behaviors that positively influence patient/client outcomes, the profession and the health needs of society.

Social Responsibility
Social responsibility is the promotion of a mutual trust between the PTA, as a member of the profession, and the larger public that necessitates responding to societal needs for health and wellness.

Evolution of the Physical Therapy Profession

In 2000, the APTA House of Delegates endorsed a vision for the profession that described the hopes for how physical therapy would be practiced in 2020 and the qualifications of those involved with PT practice. Many of the goals and outcomes associated with Vision 2020 were quite different from that of the early days of reconstruction aides, and many components of that vision have already been accomplished. Physical therapists are now being educated at the doctoral level throughout the United States, and provide services that go far beyond the traditional treatment of injury and illness to include preventive services that promote health and wellness. They most often provide their services in a manner that reflects **autonomous practice,** defined by the APTA to include exercising independent, self-determined judgment and having the ability to refer patients/clients to other health-care providers and other professionals. All jurisdictions in the United States now allow some form of **direct access** in which patients/clients are able to receive physical therapy services directly, without having to obtain a referral from another health-care provider to do so.[20] However, many third-party payers (i.e., insurance organizations such as Medicare) continue to require a physician's or other primary care provider's referral in order to cover the services provided. The APTA supports national and state-level legislative efforts to reduce the barriers for all patients seeking direct access to PT services.

In 2013, given that the profession had already met many of the internally focused goals of Vision 2020, the House of Delegates passed a new **APTA Vision Statement for Physical Therapy.** This new vision is much more externally focused, an emphasis that reflects the evolution of our profession.[21] The uniting focus in the current vision is the profession's ability to impact "movement." In describing the new vision, the APTA website explains that "movement is a key to optimal living and quality of life for all people that extends beyond health to every person's ability to participate in and contribute to society.[22] Because various systems in the human body impact movement, the APTA has defined the **movement system** as "the anatomic structures and physiologic functions that interact to move the body or its component parts."[23] In promoting the profession's specialized body of knowledge as movement experts, the APTA anticipates that physical therapy will be better poised to positively impact societal health, fitness and activity.

Vision Statement for the Physical Therapy Profession[22]

Transforming society by optimizing movement to improve the human experience.
   Guiding Principles to Achieve the Vision (see apta.org/Vision for more description)

Identity
Quality
Collaboration
Value
Innovation
Consumer-Centricity
Access/Equity
Advocacy

SUMMARY

The profession of physical therapy was developed in response to a need for health-care providers who specialized in rehabilitating those people injured or impaired by illness and disease. It has become recognized for its expertise in the area of movement dysfunction. The PTA position was created in response to a need for a formally, consistently educated, skilled health-care worker to whom PTs could confidently delegate components of physical therapy intervention. The future of physical therapist practice as "movement experts" includes using PTAs to assist in the provision of preventive and rehabilitative services to individuals who are able to access those services directly, without need of referral from another health-care provider.

REFERENCES

1. Granger FB. The development of physiotherapy. *Phys Ther.* 1976;56(1):13-14.
2. Moffat M. The history of physical therapy practice in the United States. *J Phys Ther Educ.* 2003;17(3):15-25.
3. Venes D, ed. *Taber's Encyclopedic Medical Dictionary.* 22nd ed. Philadelphia, PA: FA Davis; 2013.
4. Wojciechowski M. Celebrating a milestone: 35 years of PTAs. *PT Magazine.* 2004(2):42-49.
5. Carpenter-Davis CA. Physical therapist assistant education over the decades. *J Phys Ther Educ.* 2003;17(3):80-85.
6. Echtermach JL. The political and social issues that have shaped physical therapy education over the decades. *J Phys Ther Educ.* 2003;17(3):26-33.
7. Worthingham CA. Complimentary functions and responsibilities in an emerging profession. *Phys Ther.* 1965;45:935-939.
8. White BC. Physical therapy assistants: implications for the future. *Phys Ther.* 1970;50(5):674-679.
9. Watts NT. Task analysis and division of responsibility in physical therapy. *Phys Ther.* 1971;51(1):23-35.
10. Commission on Accreditation in Physical Therapy Education. 2012-2013 fact sheet: physical therapist assistant programs. http://www.capteonline.org/uploadedFiles/CAPTEorg/About_CAPTE/Resources/Aggregate_Program_Data/AggregateProgramData_PTAPrograms.pdf. Updated 2013. Accessed August 10, 2015.
11. American Physical Therapy Association. RC 20-12 feasibility study for transitioning to an entry-level baccalaureate physical therapist assistant degree. *2014 House of Delegates Handbook.* Fairfax, VA: American Physical Therapy Association; 2014:240-241.
12. American Physical Therapy Association. RC 02-12 feasibility study for transitioning to an entry-level baccalaureate physical therapist assistant degree: Supplemental report to 2014 House of Delegates. 2014.
13. American Physical Therapy Association. Distinction between the physical therapist and the physical therapist assistant in physical therapy (HOD

P06-01-18-19). http://www.apta.org/uploadedFiles/APTAorg/About_Us/Policies/ Terminology/DistinctionPTPTA.pdf. Updated 2012. Accessed August 10, 2015.

14. American Physical Therapy Association. Provision of physical therapy services and related tasks (HOD P06-00-17-28). http://www.apta.org/uploadedFiles/ APTAorg/About_Us/Policies/Practice/ProvisionInterventions.pdf. Updated 2012. Accessed August 10, 2015.

15. Scott RW. *Foundations of Physical Therapy.* New York, NY: McGraw-Hill; 2002:484.

16. American Physical Therapy Association. APTA to continue efforts to promote physical therapy as a distinct profession. PT in Motion News Web site. http:// www.apta.org/PTinMotion/NewsNow/2011/6/17/DistinctProfession/. Published June 17, 2011. Updated 2011. Accessed August 12, 2015.

17. Pellegrino E. What is a profession? *J Allied Health.* 1983;12(3):168.

18. American Physical Therapy Association. Professionalism in physical therapy: core values (BOD P05-04-02-03). http://www.apta.org/uploadedFiles/APTAorg/ About_Us/Policies/Judicial_Legal/ProfessionalismCoreValues.pdf. Updated 2012. Accessed August 10, 2015.

19. American Physical Therapy Association. Values-based behaviors for the physical therapist assistant. http://www.apta.org/uploadedFiles/APTAorg/About_Us/ Policies/Judicial_Legal/ValueBasedBehaviorsPTA.pdf. Updated 2013. Accessed August 10, 2015.

20. American Physical Therapy Association. Autonomous physical therapist practice: definitions and privileges (BOD P03-03-12-28). http://www.apta.org/ uploadedFiles/APTAorg/About_Us/Policies/Practice/AutonomousPTPractice DefinitionsPrivileges.pdf. Updated 2012. Accessed August 10, 2015.

21. Purtilo R. A time to harvest, a time to sow: ethics for a shifting landscape. *Phys Ther.* 2000;80(11):1112-1119.

22. American Physical Therapy Association. Vision statement for the physical therapy profession and guiding principles to achieve the vision. http:// www.apta.org/Vision/. Updated 2015. Accessed August 10, 2015.

23. American Physical Therapy Association. Definition of movement system: Report to the 2015 House of Delegates. *2015 House of Delegates Handbook.* Fairfax, VA: American Physical Therapy Association; 2015:49.

Name _____

REVIEW

1. Describe two different historical events that led to the creation and evolution of the physical therapy profession. Why were these events significant?

_____

_____

_____

_____

_____

_____

2. When was the PTA position officially created by the APTA? List at least two factors that led to the creation of a new health-care provider position.

_____

_____

_____

_____

_____

3. Using the criteria developed by Watts and reviewed in Chapter 1, list and describe four factors that a PT should use in determining the tasks that could be performed by a PTA.

_____

_____

_____

_____

_____

(questions continue on page 16)

Application

1. Review the APTA documents "Professionalism in Physical Therapy: Core Values" and "Values-Based Behaviors for the PTA." For each of the behaviors listed below, give one example of how it might be demonstrated by a physical therapist assistant.

Values-Based Behavior	How It Is Demonstrated by a PTA
Altruism	
Caring/Compassion	
Continuing Competence	
Duty	
Integrity	
PT/PTA Collaboration	
Responsibility	
Social Responsibility	

2. The APTA's vision statement is "Transforming Society by Optimizing Movement to Improve the Human Experience." How does this relate to your desire to become a physical therapist assistant? How do you see yourself living this vision?

2

Physical Therapist Practice Settings

CHAPTER OBJECTIVES

After reading this chapter, the reader will be able to:

- Give examples of activities and techniques that physical therapists (PTs) and physical therapist assistants (PTAs) use to help an individual improve movement skills and achieve maximum functional ability.
- Describe the purpose of the American Physical Therapy Association's (APTA's) *Guide to Physical Therapist Practice.*
- Explain how the International Classification of Functioning, Disability and Health model is used as a tool for individualizing each patient's needs, goals, and interventions.
- Describe typical practice settings in which PTs and PTAs are employed.
- Identify common patient conditions seen and interventions provided by PTs and PTAs in typical practice settings.
- Describe how PTAs are utilized in various practice settings and with different patient populations.
- List other professions and health-care providers with whom PTs and PTAs most commonly interact.

KEY TERMS AND CONCEPTS

- *Guide to Physical Therapist Practice*
- International Classification of Functioning, Disability and Health
- Acute care
- Outpatient
- Skilled nursing/extended care/transitional care facility
- Home care
- Hospice
- Pediatrics
- Floating/traveling PT
- Academia
- Interprofessional Education

Jamal and May have just started their first year of a PTA program. As they get to know each other, they talk about what got them interested in physical therapy. Jamal describes how he learned about physical therapy when his grandmother broke her hip. "She couldn't come home from the hospital until she went to a skilled nursing facility for physical therapy and to get stronger." May tells Jamal about her experience with physical therapy in the outpatient setting. "Could I work in a clinic like that if I am a PTA?" asks Jamal. May says, "I think PTAs can work anywhere that a PT does . . . their role is just a little bit different, depending on the setting and the patients they see."

QUESTIONS TO CONSIDER

In addition to outpatient clinics and skilled nursing facilities, in what other types of settings do PTs and PTAs work? What types of services do they provide in each setting? Do PTAs have different responsibilities in different settings? Who else works with PTs and PTAs?

Chapter 1 covers how PT practice began and how it grew to include the PTA. This chapter discusses the most common practice settings in which PTs and PTAs are employed. Before doing so, however, it will be helpful to see how physical therapy is currently delivered, regardless of practice setting.

Current PT Practice

PTs identify themselves as "the experts in the analysis of human movement, performance, and function."[1] In very general terms, the focus of PT practice (which, as stated in Chapter 1, includes the PTA as the sole individual who can assist the PT in the delivery of physical therapy services) is to maximize an individual's functional ability by improving his movement skills. Enabling someone to achieve maximum functional ability is often accomplished by:

- Reducing pain, inflammation, and/or muscle tightness
- Improving strength, joint mobility, coordination, and flexibility
- Increasing cardiopulmonary function and endurance
- Promoting an intact integumentary system via wound care, prevention of scarring, or the application of physical agents to encourage circulation and healing
- Educating the patient on safety, prevention of illness and injury, and health/wellness strategies
- Teaching the patient new movement techniques to avoid repetitive-type injuries or to compensate for movement capability lost due to injury or illness

How do clinicians decide which interventions are most important for each person to whom they provide services? One tool that helps define the process is the ***Guide to Physical Therapist Practice.*** The *Guide*, as it is commonly called, was originally published in 1997 and then revised in 2001 and again in 2014. The first two hard-copy versions were designed to be used as resources to educate those outside of physical therapy about the services that PT could provide. However, because those outside the profession most likely now use other resources to learn about physical therapy, version 3.0 has been revised as a description of current practice for PTs and PTAs and has been converted to an online-only document that now may be updated easily and more frequently in order to provide the most current practice information.[2]

The *Guide* differentiates between patients and clients, two different groups who may benefit from physical therapy services (refer to the preface of this textbook for information on how the term "patient" is used in this text). The *Guide* also describes the types of conditions seen in physical therapy and the many types of tests, measures, and interventions used by clinicians to treat those conditions. Within their patient/client management responsibilities, physical therapists assess the patient's current status and make determinations of her potential for improvement, based on tests and measures used as part of their examinations and evaluations. Chapter 3 describes the process of patient/client management and the PTA's role within it in greater detail.

The *Guide to Physical Therapist Practice* defines the terms "patients" and "clients" in the following manner:[2]

Patients: Individuals who are the recipients of physical therapy examination, evaluation, diagnosis, prognosis, and intervention and who have a disease, disorder, condition, impairment, functional limitation, or disability.

Clients: Individuals who engage the services of a physical therapist and who can benefit from the physical therapist's consultation, interventions, professional advice, health promotion, fitness, wellness, or prevention services. Clients are also businesses, school systems, and others to whom physical therapists provide services.

Reprinted with permission of the American Physical Therapy Association from the *Guide to Physical Therapist Practice 3.0*, available at http://guidetoptpractice.apta.org. Accessed December 30, 2015. This material is copyrighted, and any further reproduction or distribution requires written permission from APTA.

The most recent edition of the *Guide* now encourages clinicians to consider a new patient classification model as part of the process of developing patient/client goals and intervention strategies. In 2008, the APTA House of Delegates voted to accept the World Health Organization's **International Classification of Functioning, Disability and Health** (ICF) model of patient categorization (Fig. 2-1).[3] In this model, health and disability are classified in a manner that is not mutually exclusive; each person's biopsychosocial (physical, psychological, and societal) response to a given health condition will affect his level of function differently. The focus,

Interaction Among the Components of the International Classification of Functioning, Disability and Health (ICF) Model of Functioning and Disability

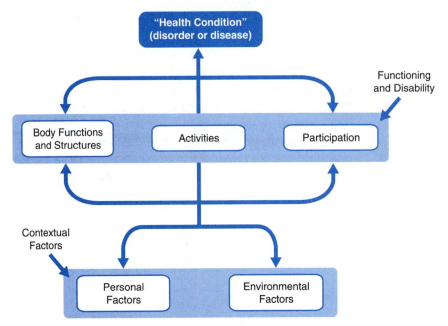

Figure 2-1. Diagram of ICF Model Components, as Defined by the World Health Organization. (From the *Guide to Physical Therapist Practice, Version 3.0.*)

therefore, should be less on the condition and more on the impact of the associated functional loss on one's activities and ability to participate in society.[4] The ICF's model of disability also encourages health-care providers to consider in greater depth the personal and environmental factors that can also cause one person's response to functional loss to be very different from that of another person's, even if their physiological levels of function are similar.

FOR REFLECTION

■ Identify a health condition that may be addressed by physical therapy. Can you think of ways in which one person with that health condition might present differently from another person with that same condition? What factors might influence those differences?

The use of ICF language and concepts allows the emphasis to be focused on the patient's capabilities and current functional status rather than on those abilities that may have been lost or altered.[4] Identifying an individual patient's abilities, limitations, and restrictions can be used to focus an intervention session more specifically on that patient's unique needs, and can also provide helpful terminology for developing and documenting the status of patient goals.

Key Phrases Used in ICF Terminology

Body Functions: physiological functions of body systems (including psychological functions).

Body Structures: anatomical parts of the body such as organs, limbs and their components.

Impairments: problems in body function or structure such as a significant deviation or loss.

Activity: the execution of a task or action by an individual.

Participation: involvement in a life situation.

Activity Limitations: difficulties an individual may have in executing activities.

Participation Restrictions: problems an individual may experience in involvement in life situations.

Environmental Factors: the physical, social and attitudinal environment in which people live and conduct their lives

Reprinted with permission of the World Health Organization, from "Towards a Common Language for Functioning, Disability and Health," available at http://www.who.int/classifications/icf/en/. Accessed December 30, 2015.

Physical Therapy Clinical Settings

PTAs work in most of the same practice settings and with most of the same types of patients as do PTs. The specific tasks and interventions performed, as well as the level of supervision required or requested, vary depending on the setting or by state law (see Chapter 4) and by the use of Watts's criteria for direction and supervision (see Chapter 1). However, there are many common features of a PTA's scope of work relative to a given practice setting. The most common settings in which PTAs are employed are the following:

Acute care
Outpatient
Skilled nursing facilities (SNFs), extended care facilities (ECFs), transitional care units (TCUs), and subacute rehabilitation facilities
Home care/hospice
Pediatric specialty clinics
Agencies providing **floating/traveling PT services**
Academia

Acute Care Physical Therapy

PTAs may provide physical therapy services within the physical therapy department of a hospital setting or see patients at bedside (within their rooms). Any hospitalized patient may require physical therapy. However, those who most often receive services are patients who have:

- Injuries related to a fall (for example, a patient who sustains a hip fracture) or a need for surgery (emergency or planned) on joints, bones, or major organs
- An exacerbation (flare-up) of a chronic illness, such as chronic obstructive pulmonary disease, congestive heart failure, or cancer
- Acute conditions such as pneumonia, influenza, or a urinary tract infection
- Weakness due to chronic or multiple medical conditions
- Severe pain from an unknown source or pain that cannot be adequately controlled by medication

Physical therapy in the acute care setting frequently focuses on improving the patient's strength, endurance, and tolerance for being out of bed, progressing to more advanced functional mobility activities as the patient's abilities allow. The goal is often to enable patients to return home or to a lesser level of care, although more physical therapy may still be needed after the patient has been discharged to maximize the patient's functional abilities.

Specialized areas of physical therapy include several within the acute care settings:

- *Cardiac rehabilitation:* Patients are seen as inpatients or outpatients in relation to decreased functional capacity following hospitalization for heart vessel bypass surgery, valve repair, or myocardial infarction (heart attack). Cardiac rehabilitation may also be used with at-risk patients to minimize the likelihood of a cardiac-related event occurring in the future.
- *Inpatient rehabilitation:* Especially in larger hospitals, those patients who sustain a significant neuromuscular event such as a cerebrovascular accident (stroke) may be placed in an inpatient rehabilitation (IPR) unit. Other neurological diagnoses seen in an IPR unit include traumatic brain or closed head injuries, spinal cord injuries, tumors of the central nervous system, or acute, chronic, or progressive neurological diseases such as Guillain-Barré syndrome, multiple sclerosis, or Parkinson disease. Patients seen in the IPR setting may also have multiple medical conditions or complications, such as multiple fractures sustained in a motor vehicle accident or a lower-extremity amputation as a result of a diabetic foot ulcer. IPR physical therapy often focuses on improving gross mobility levels, such as rolling and getting into or out of bed, transferring in and out of a wheelchair, and ambulation, with or without the use of assistive devices or braces. Patients with severe neurological conditions may not be able to return completely to their previous level of physical mobility. In such cases, the goals of physical therapy are to help patients learn and adapt to different ways of moving, with assistive equipment as needed, to obtain maximum functional ability.
- *Wound care:* PTs, and to a lesser extent PTAs, may be involved in the application of hydrotherapy or electrotherapy to encourage wound healing. Depending on the practice regulations in a given state, PTs may also recommend and/or apply wound dressings or perform sharp wound debridement. PTAs may assist with the application of interventions and dressings, but sharp débridement is one skill that

the APTA considers appropriate only for PTs to perform.[5] The topic of interventions that should be performed exclusively by PTs is addressed in Chapter 9.

- *Emergency room physical therapy:* An emerging area of practice within acute care is physical therapy provided in the emergency room setting. Patients may need instruction on how to care for acute musculoskeletal injuries, how to use assistive devices such as crutches, or how to perform preventive exercises or mobility techniques that will allow them to maintain function while avoiding further injury. Owing to the one-time-only nature of these visits, physical therapy in this type of setting is almost exclusively provided by PTs.

FOR REFLECTION
FOR REFLECTION

- Which area of physical therapy in the acute care setting would be most challenging for you? Why?

Outpatient Physical Therapy

According to the APTA, the private practice outpatient clinic employed the highest percentage of APTA-member PTAs compared with other settings. When combined with those PTAs employed in hospital-based outpatient facilities, this setting provides employment for approximately half the APTA's PTA members.[6] This may not be representative of all PTAs because not all PTAs are APTA members. However, the U.S. Department of Labor's most recent statistics also indicate that the outpatient setting is the most common employment setting for PTAs.[7]

In the typical outpatient setting, PTs and PTAs are likely to work with patients with a variety of musculoskeletal and, less commonly, neuromuscular disorders. Common diagnoses seen in this setting include musculoskeletal strains and sprains or inflammatory injuries such as tendinitis and bursitis, often related to overuse. Patients may also be seen following fractures, after surgeries such as a rotator cuff or meniscus repair, or after a joint replacement. The age range of patients seen in the outpatient setting goes from school-age children to the geriatric (older adult) population. Patients are usually living independently, although not necessarily alone, and usually do not need to receive therapy on a daily basis. Patients seen by PTAs are frequently instructed in exercises to improve strength, flexibility, balance, or posture that are to be performed at home independently or with the assistance of a family member. These are referred to as home exercise programs (HEPs). The patient returns to physical therapy for periodic revision of the HEP to continue making optimal progress. Modalities such as hot packs, cold packs, ultrasound, mechanical traction, and electrical stimulation may be used to control pain and edema or to reduce muscle spasm.

Many types of specialized outpatient clinics work with specific diagnoses or types of patients. Many outpatient therapists specialize in manual therapy, which involves the application of mobilizing or manipulative forces on soft tissue or joint structures. Some of the techniques used in manual therapy, such as spinal and joint

mobilization, are considered by the APTA to be outside of the PTA's scope of work.[5]
Other specialized areas of outpatient practice include the following:

- *Sports medicine:* Clinicians may work with athletes in general, or their work may
  be specific to one type of sport or athlete. PTs and PTAs at these clinics may work
  with athletic trainers, may have strengthening/conditioning certifications, or may be
  dually qualified in physical therapy and athletic training. It is not uncommon for
  clinicians with dual training to work with local high school or college teams to
  provide services during practices or games in addition to providing traditional
  clinic services.
- *Gender health/women's health:* Clinicians treat conditions that are unique to or that
  present differently in different genders, such as incontinence, pelvic floor
  dysfunction, or certain types of athletic issues.
- *Aquatic therapy:* PTs and PTAs work with patients who perform exercises, usually
  in a swimming pool, with the assistance or resistance provided by water.
- *Industrial medicine:* PTs and PTAs analyze on-the-job task performance, often in
  the patient's work environment, to determine ways that repetitive trauma can be
  minimized while allowing maximum comfort and efficiency.
- *Performing arts therapy:* Clinicians work with actors, dancers, and/or musicians to
  deal with their unique injuries related to performance and practice.

FOR REFLECTION

- Many students are interested in physical therapy because of an experience
  they (or someone they knew) had in the outpatient setting. If that applies to
  you, describe to a classmate how that experience fostered your interest in
  physical therapy.

SNFs, ECFs, TCUs, and Subacute Rehabilitation Facilities

Skilled nursing facilities (SNFs), extended care facilities (ECFs), transitional care
units (TCUs), and subacute rehabilitation facilities are terms that describe the
different types of residential and rehabilitative units available for older adults,
patients with chronic medical needs, and/or patients who need ongoing rehabilitation
prior to returning to a more independent living setting.

SNFs provide residential and medical services for adults (primarily older adults)
who require 24-hour medical care, constant supervision for safety, or extensive
assistance with mobility. The term "nursing home" was formerly used to describe
this type of setting. The person who lives here is called a "resident" rather than a
"patient" to indicate respect for the fact that the facility has become the person's
home. Any resident may receive physical therapy if there is a documented loss of
functional ability and a reasonable expectation of improvement. This is most often
justified if there has been a precipitating event, such as an acute musculoskeletal,
neuromuscular, or cardiopulmonary injury or illness, that has led to a change in
status. However, at any given time most permanent residents of an SNF are not
receiving physical therapy.

Within the SNF, there may be specific units designed for patients who have recently been hospitalized but who need further short-term rehabilitative services before returning home or to a lesser level of care, such as an assisted living facility. These short-term-stay units are often called ECFs, TCUs, or subacute rehabilitation units. For this chapter, the abbreviation TCU is used to describe all three of these settings.

In the TCU, most patients need orders for daily physical, occupational, and/or speech therapy as a criterion for being admitted. They may be guaranteed only a certain number of days before being required to move to another unit or facility. The patient's ability to stay in the TCU is generally dependent on the need for daily skilled services and the ability to demonstrate improvement, but the length of stay can also be affected by the patient's willingness to participate and his overall medical status.

Many of the patients seen for physical therapy in the TCU often have multiple medical conditions. However, any patient admitted to a TCU is admitted under the assumption that the placement is short term. Patients may be admitted for any of the same reasons that would cause them to be admitted to an acute care facility. It is almost routine for elderly patients to be admitted to a TCU following a cerebrovascular accident or after surgery for a total hip or total knee arthroplasty. Many of the injuries sustained by those admitted to TCUs are related to falls. These include hip fractures, upper-extremity fractures (often sustained when a patient lands on an outstretched hand), head trauma including contusions and concussions, and vertebral compression fractures (which can also occur unrelated to a fall). A patient who falls and is unable to get up may lie on the floor for an extended period before help arrives. These patients may be further deconditioned, dehydrated, or have areas of skin breakdown because of this prolonged immobility.

Other patients may also arrive deconditioned due to a prolonged hospitalization for such cardiopulmonary conditions as pneumonia or congestive heart failure. Even though the medical condition may be under control, the prolonged inactivity or bedrest associated with the illness may have led to severe weakness or functional mobility deficits. Occasionally, patients may be admitted without a specific diagnosis but with an unexplained history of falling, back pain, or weakness associated with weight loss. This last condition is often referred to as a "failure to thrive" and may be related to cognitive deficits or depression leading to poor nutritional intake.[8]

The PTA working in these types of settings often focuses on maximizing the resident's mobility skills. In the TCU, the goals often include independent bed mobility/transfer skills and independent ambulation with some type of assistive device, such as a walker. At this point, the patient often is mobile enough to return to the previous living setting but may require additional physical therapy on a home care or outpatient basis to progress to a less restrictive assistive device, such as a cane, or no device at all. Other interventions commonly used include therapeutic exercises to promote range of motion, increase strength and functional activity tolerance, or improve balance and coordination. Functional activities such as car or toilet transfers may be practiced, and caregivers (staff, family members, or friends) may be trained in how to assist the patient with these activities. Ambulation may be practiced on various surfaces, such as carpet, a sidewalk, or stairs. Gait and balance abilities may be assessed to determine whether a patient is at future risk of falling, using standardized functional tests such as the Berg Balance Scale or the Dynamic Gait Index. Most clinicians agree that a PTA can administer the components of these tests, although the PT should interpret the results. Physical agents may be used to facilitate stretching of stiff joint and muscle tissue, to relieve pain, to control edema, or to promote wound healing.

FOR REFLECTION

- Many PTAs find work after graduation in the TCU type of setting. Do you think you would like working with the elderly population? Why or why not? Compare your answer with those of your classmates.

Home Care

Many patients who live independently may require physical therapy services but have limited ability to access outpatient services because of mobility limitations or medical conditions. These clients (the term more often used in referring to home care recipients, again in deference to their living situation) may qualify for physical therapy services provided in the home. The PT must first determine whether the client meets the criteria (most often set by the client's insurance provider) for receiving home care services. Merely being unable to drive or lacking transportation to an outpatient clinic is not enough justification for receiving physical therapy in the home. However, for many clients who are considered "homebound," physical therapy can play an integral part in progressing them to a more mobile status that allows them to eventually leave their home with greater ease. For those clients who have more permanent mobility deficits, home care physical therapy may enable them to maximize and retain their highest level of function, enabling them to stay in an independent or assisted living setting versus having to move to an SNF.

Because of the high costs of living permanently in an SNF, some clients living in an independent or assisted living setting will elect to sign on to ongoing physical therapy services, even if such services are not covered under insurance. They are willing to pay the full costs of these services in the belief that regular, ongoing therapy will enable them to maintain their current functional levels for as long as possible. It is hoped that this will delay or prevent a future move to an SNF, adding to their quality of life while minimizing their expenses in the long run.

In addition to working with the client, home care clinicians also often work with family members, friends, or other caregivers to instruct them in exercise techniques or in how they might best assist the client with mobility tasks. Caregivers may require instruction in proper body mechanics to avoid physical injury and may need to be connected with social workers or other health-care professionals who can provide resources for psychosocial support, as those who serve as a caregiver to a dependent family member often report high levels of stress.[9]

Because of the independent nature of home care physical therapy, a PTA (or PT) who works in this type of setting is usually expected to have had prior experience working more directly with other clinicians in more traditional settings of service delivery. The PTA working in home care has to comply with all of the supervisory regulations that apply in that particular state and setting (see Chapter 4) but generally will be at the client's home without a PT or other health-care provider present. Because of the variable nature of the clients and the environments in which they live, home care PTAs have to recognize changes in the client's status that might warrant consultation with a PT, other providers involved with that client's care, or an immediate 911 call. This ability for quick assessment and decision-making often requires significant experience with patients and other clinicians.

A home care clinician requires high levels of creativity and problem-solving ability. He has to use a variety of exercises, often improvising or revising the plan for a given therapy session based on the equipment available, the client's willingness to participate, or a new client concern. Therefore, the clinician must have had ample opportunity to build his repertoire of appropriate PT exercises and activities. In addition, the home care clinician often needs to have special interpersonal skills. Often, clients seen in their own home may feel entitled to direct the therapy session more than they might in the "medical" environment of an acute care hospital or SNF. They may want to treat the home care clinician as a "guest" in their home and may not understand the importance of staying on task or beginning and ending the therapy session at a prearranged time. Sometimes they may ask the clinician to help them with household tasks or other activities unrelated to the therapy session. Therefore, the clinician needs to have strong time management skills and the ability to keep control of the PT session in a way that still respects the client's needs and wishes.

Hospice

Patients who have terminal illnesses, such as cancer, who most likely have fewer than 6 months to live (as determined by a physician), and who are no longer receiving ongoing treatment to "cure" their diagnosis can receive a multitude of health-care services through hospice care. Most patients receive hospice services in their homes, although they may also receive them in SNFs, assisted living settings, special hospice facilities, or hospice units in acute care hospitals.

Why would someone diagnosed with a terminal illness be appropriate for rehabilitation services? When first seeing a patient, the evaluating PT always establishes a physical therapy diagnosis, which is separate from the patient's medical diagnosis (more information about this process is found in Chapter 3). The PT then establishes a prognosis (an expectation for improvement) related to the physical therapy diagnosis. It is not unusual in hospice care (and sometimes in other settings) that, even though the patient's overall prognosis is poor or terminal, he does have potential for improving an activity limitation or participation restriction that will then enable the patient to maximize his quality of life during the time left to live.

A common example of how this occurs can be seen with the intervention of transfer training. A patient who undergoes exploratory surgery that results in a diagnosis of cancer with a terminal prognosis may require a prolonged hospital stay to stabilize his medical condition. He may then return home under hospice care in an extremely weakened state, needing extensive assistance for transferring to and from the bed and the toilet. If the patient can participate in strengthening exercises and transfer training to help improve his mobility, it will enable him to maintain as much independence as possible and ease the burden on his caregivers (which often affects the patient's ability to stay at home). Minimizing the patient's need for reliance on others may also improve his overall psychological status. Working to train the caregivers to help the patient, when he does require more physical assistance, may enable the patient to avoid prolonged bedrest and maintain a better quality of life. Many patients receiving hospice services hope to remain at home for the entire end-of-life process, and a patient who requires less physical assistance with mobility probably has a better chance of achieving that goal.

Another common focus of hospice care is to treat physical or psychosocial causes of pain or discomfort. This is also referred to as palliative care, though palliative care can be provided to any patient in any stage of illness, not just those in hospice.[10] Physical therapy can contribute to palliative care via the use of physical agents such as heat, as well as through exercises, massage, or other manual therapy techniques that may ease musculoskeletal restrictions or imbalances causing pain or discomfort.

Pediatrics

Many students enter a PTA program with a goal of someday working in the area of pediatric physical therapy. Students with this goal must recognize the complexity of dealing with the impairments and disabilities that children have as a result of acute, chronic, permanent, or progressive illnesses or disorders. Dealing with these impairments becomes even more challenging when a child lacks the maturity or cognitive ability to understand the nature of the illness or the ability to participate fully in his therapy.

Although children can sustain many of the same types of acute musculoskeletal injuries as adults, their impairments are more likely the result of chronic neuromuscular diseases or disorders. They may be caused by birth defects (such as in spina bifida), a birth or early childhood injury that might lead to cerebral palsy, or inherited disorders or other genetically related conditions, such as Down syndrome, cystic fibrosis, or muscular dystrophy. The deficits seen may also be the result of poor prenatal practices on the part of the child's mother, such as in fetal alcohol syndrome, or caused by abusive behavior by a parent or caregiver, as occurs in shaken baby syndrome. Cancers or nonmalignant tumors, blood diseases, near drowning, and closed head injuries can also leave children with significant ongoing functional deficits.

Physical therapy in the pediatric setting is often focused on maximizing the child's motor control and overall functional mobility level by improving strength, flexibility, balance, and coordination. Physical therapy may also involve techniques that use sensory input to increase the child's awareness of his surroundings or to help him respond more appropriately to normal stimulation occurring within the environment.[11] Through tasks that may seem like play to the untrained eye, the PT or PTA engages the child in developmentally based activities specifically designed to facilitate or inhibit an imbalance in neuromuscular activity. As in the home care setting, the clinicians have to demonstrate high levels of creativity, an ability to change activities quickly based on the child's response, and the skill to keep the child "on task." Pediatric clinicians must be especially responsive to these children's nonverbal messages because they may have limited ability to communicate verbally.

Because the child does not always understand why the activities are important and may be resistant to them, the pediatric clinician must work closely with the child's parents and other caregivers. They must be taught to understand the necessity for and goals of the child's physical therapy program because they are often responsible for assisting with mobility tasks and for ensuring follow-through. Many parents may not be realistic about their child's ability to improve, and the therapist must encourage their full participation in therapy without giving them false hope.

Because of the chronic or progressive nature of many of the diagnoses seen with this population, pediatric physical therapy also has to focus on prevention. Manual therapy, stretching, and bracing are often used to prevent contractures (loss of joint motion caused by severe connective tissue shortening) that would further reduce the child's mobility. Aggressive exercises to stretch or strengthen may be used after surgical or chemical release of contractures to regain range of motion and prevent recurrence. Equipment such as ambulation assistive devices or wheelchairs may need special adaptation and periodic revision because of the child's growth or improvement or decline in the child's abilities. Because many of these children require adaptive equipment and ongoing skilled medical services for a lifetime, PTs and PTAs working in this setting often need special advocacy skills. By thoroughly presenting the needs of their clients to other medical care providers or organizations, insurance companies, or state and federal government agencies, the PT or PTA can help the child's parents obtain as many needed services as possible.

PTs and PTAs who work with the pediatric population may do so in a number of different settings. Traditional acute care facilities may have a separate pediatric unit, but there are also acute care hospitals that see children exclusively. Outpatient clinics may see children as a portion of their full outpatient clientele, but children who need ongoing services related to chronic illnesses or injuries will often receive them at an outpatient facility that specializes in pediatrics. Children of school age may also receive physical therapy services within the school system. The Individuals with Disabilities Educational Act (IDEA) is a federal law that allows children with disabilities improved access to a public school education through the provision of specialized services, which often includes physical therapy. Instead of the traditional physical therapy plan of care, children receiving services in school have an "individualized educational plan," an interdisciplinary document that addresses each child's specific physical, psychosocial, and educational needs.[12] PTs and PTAs work with other disciplines to maximize the child's ability to participate in the educational process to give him the best chance for independence, employment, and socialization in adulthood.[13]

FOR REFLECTION

- In your opinion, what would be the most challenging aspect of working in a pediatric setting?

Because of the complexity of many of the conditions and intervention techniques used with the pediatric population, in addition to the highly developed interpersonal skills required in dealing with children and their parents, it is unusual (although not impossible) for a newly graduated PTA to obtain a position in pediatrics. Most clinics require that PTAs (and even PTs) have some experience in more traditional physical therapy settings before progressing to pediatrics.

Floating/Traveling PTA

Some PTAs choose to work for agencies or facilities that use PTAs in a variety of settings and locations. Some are similar types of facilities within a limited geographic area, and the work location may change daily, a process called "floating." Other organizations may provide staffing for a variety of facility types located across a larger geographic region or even throughout the country, with assignments for these "traveling" (temporary) employees lasting weeks or months. A floating or traveling PTA must be flexible, enjoy a variety of responsibilities, catch on quickly to new routines, and work comfortably in different settings under variable levels and styles of supervision. Employers usually prefer that PTAs taking a floating/traveling position have experience in more traditional employment formats before beginning this type of work.

Academia

Some PTAs work on college campuses in PTA (and occasionally doctor of physical therapy) educational programs. Depending on the requirements of the institution, PTAs may function as faculty assistants, or they may be a primary faculty member responsible for classroom content or clinical placements. PTAs who have obtained a master's degree are also qualified to serve as the director of a PTA program. Many PTAs (as well as PTs) who work in academia will also continue to work in the clinical environment, especially during times when the academic program is not in session. They are often actively engaged in research activities related to their clinical or teaching expertise. Chapter 14 explores how PTAs interested in teaching or research might prepare themselves for that type of special career opportunity.

Interacting With Other Health-Care Professionals

In most practice settings, PTs and PTAs will interact with a variety of other health-care professionals. They may work side by side in a department, interact at patient care conferences or via the medical record, or work together only when needs arise that are outside of the physical therapist scope of practice. The other health-care providers and professionals with whom physical therapy clinicians will interact most often fall into these general, nonexclusive categories:

- Other traditional rehabilitation providers, such as occupational therapists and speech-language pathologists
- Those who provide some services that are similar to those provided by physical therapy, including athletic trainers, personal trainers, chiropractors, massage therapists, acupuncturists, and exercise physiologists
- Those who provide ongoing direct care to the patient, including physicians and physician assistants, nurses and nursing staff, pharmacists, psychologists, and dentists
- Clinicians who interact with patients on a one-time or less frequent basis, such as radiography and sonography technicians, respiratory therapists, phlebotomists, prosthetists, or orthotists
- Professionals who interact with the patient in a non-hands-on manner to meet their medical or psychosocial needs, including social workers, dietitians, health information managers, chaplains, and holistic health providers

PTAs must have a working knowledge and appreciation of those other disciplines in order to best work together in meeting patients' needs. In these times of limitations to payment for services, it has become even more critical for disciplines to communicate and collaborate in order to prioritize and avoid duplication of services. To promote this expectation, in 2014 the APTA's House of Delegates endorsed competencies for interprofessional interaction as developed by the Interprofessional Education Collaborative, a group representing multiple health-care provider groups.[14]

Interprofessional Collaborative Practice Competencies[15]

1. Values/Ethics for Interprofessional Practice: Work with individuals of other professions to maintain a climate of mutual respect and shared values.
2. Roles/Responsibilities: Use the knowledge of one's own role and those of other professions to appropriately assess and address the health-care needs of the patients and populations served.
3. Interprofessional Communication: Communicate with patients, families, communities, and other health professionals in a responsive and responsible manner that supports a team approach to the maintenance of health and the treatment of disease.
4. Teams and Teamwork: Apply relationship-building values and the principles of team dynamics to perform effectively in different team roles to plan and deliver patient-/population-centered care that is safe, timely, efficient, effective, and equitable.

These interprofessional education competencies are now being addressed and reinforced within many physical therapy programs via case-based tutorials that bring several groups of students from various disciplines together to discuss how they would interact with a given patient and one another, in teaming students from various disciplines together during clinicals, or by the use of on- or off-campus clinics where students and faculty from multiple professions work together in providing patient care.

FOR REFLECTION

- What other health-care programs are offered at your educational institution? With which ones would you be most likely to interact in the clinical setting? Are there non-health-care fields of study at your institution with which you might interact as a PTA?

SUMMARY

The services that PTs and PTAs provide in any setting are based on each patient's individual functional losses, activity limitations and participation restrictions, and environmental or personal factors that might influence the patient's ability to achieve his goals. PTs and PTAs work in most of the same settings, although their roles and responsibilities differ. These settings include acute care facilities, SNFs and TCUs, outpatient clinics, home care, hospice, those settings specializing in pediatric care, and academia. In nearly every setting, the PT/PTA team will work with other health-care providers and professionals. To develop a deeper knowledge and higher comfort level in interacting with other disciplines, many academic programs have embraced the concept of interprofessional education wherein students are able to work together to develop skills in collaboration, in order to most effectively meet the needs and best interests of the patient/client.

REFERENCES

1. American Physical Therapy Association. Americans with disabilities: role of the American Physical Therapy Association in advocacy, promotion, and accommodation (HOD P06-04-12-12). http://www.apta.org/uploadedFiles/APTAorg/About_Us/Policies/Health_Social_Environment/AmericansWithDisabilities.pdf. Updated 2012. Accessed July 6, 2015.
2. American Physical Therapy Association. *Guide to Physical Therapist Practice 3.0*. Alexandria, VA: American Physical Therapy Association. http://guidetoptpractice.apta.org/. Updated 2014. Accessed July 6, 2015.
3. American Physical Therapy Association. Endorsement of International Classification of Functioning, Disability and Health (ICF) (HOD P06-08-11-04). http://www.apta.org/uploadedFiles/APTAorg/About_Us/Policies/Practice/EndorsementICF.pdf. Updated 2012. Accessed July 6, 2015.
4. World Health Organization. International Classification of Functioning, Disability and Health (ICF). http://www.who.int/classifications/icf/en/. Updated 2014. Accessed July 6, 2015.
5. American Physical Therapy Association. Procedural interventions exclusively performed by physical therapists (HOD P06-00-30-36). http://www.apta.org/uploadedFiles/APTAorg/About_Us/Policies/Practice/ProceduralInterventions.pdf. Updated 2012. Accessed July 6, 2015.

6. American Physical Therapy Association. Demographic profile of physical therapist assistant members. http://www.apta.org/PTA/Careers/. Updated 2010. Accessed July 6, 2015.

7. US Department of Labor. Physical therapist assistants: occupational employment and wages, May 2014. Bureau of Labor Statistics Website. http://www.bls.gov/oes/current/oes312021.htm. Updated 2015. Accessed July 6, 2015.

8. Venes D, ed. *Taber's Encyclopedic Medical Dictionary*. 22nd ed. Philadelphia, PA: FA Davis; 2013.

9. Schulz R, Sherwood PR. Physical and mental health effects of family caregiving. *Am J Nurs*. 2008;108:23-27.

10. U.S. National Library of Medicine. What is palliative care? MedLine Plus Website. https://www.nlm.nih.gov/medlineplus/ency/patientinstructions/000536.htm. Updated 2014. Accessed December 30, 2015.

11. Chapman D, Porter RE. Sensory considerations in therapeutic interventions. In: Connolly BH, Montgomery PC, eds. *Therapeutic Exercise in Developmental Disabilities*. 3rd ed. Thorofare, NJ: SLACK; 2005:547.

12. U.S. Department of Education. Building the legacy: IDEA 2004. http://idea.ed.gov/. Updated 2013. Accessed July 6, 2015.

13. Bohmert JA. Physical therapy in the educational environment. In: Connolly BH, Montgomery PC, eds. *Therapeutic Exercise in Developmental Disabilities*. 3rd ed. Thorofare, NJ: SLACK; 2005.

14. American Physical Therapy Association. Endorsement of Interprofessional Education Collaborative Core Competencies. http://www.apta.org/uploadedFiles/APTAorg/About_Us/Policies/Education/EndordementofInterprofessional%20Education.pdf. Updated 2014. Accessed July, 2015.

15. Interprofessional Education Collaborative. Interprofessional Collaborative Practice Competencies. https://ipecollaborative.org/uploads/IP-Collaborative-Practice-Core-Competencies.pdf. Updated 2011. Accessed July 1, 2015.

Name _____

REVIEW

1. Using the following table, identify one type of *patient health condition* with which you might work and one *physical therapy intervention technique* that you might provide in each of the following settings:

Setting	Health Condition	Intervention Techniques
Acute care		
Outpatient		
SNF/ECF/TCU		
Home care/hospice		
Pediatrics		

2. Why do those PTAs who work in the home care/hospice setting or as a traveling/floating PTA often need to have more experience before beginning work in those settings?

_____

_____

_____

_____

3. Along with PT, which two professions have historically been considered part of the traditional rehabilitation department?

_____

_____

_____

_____

(questions continue on page 36)

Application

1. Terry is a high school teacher and football coach who underwent surgery for a benign brain tumor. He is now unable to walk long distances or stand for long periods because of fatigue, weakness, and balance issues. He has returned to teaching but is unable to coach his team during games because of difficulty in maneuvering his wheelchair through the grass and the crowded sidelines of the football field. He is very motivated to continue coaching, but his wife thinks he should resign his position so that he has more quality time with his family. Using the ICF model found in Figure 2-1, give two examples of the each of the following:

   a. Body Structures/Functions affected by this condition.

   b. Activity limitations and participation restrictions as a result of his condition.

   c. Environmental and personal factors that could influence his recovery.

2. Choose one of the professions that you identified as a potential interprofessional team member in the preceding question, and find out more about that profession. What is the level of education within that profession? Are there different roles or levels of education (e.g., PT and PTA) within that profession? What is that profession's main area of focus in terms of patient goals and interventions? Do they provide interventions that potentially overlap with PT?

3. After reading the descriptions of the various practice settings in which PTAs may work, identify the one(s) in which you see yourself most likely to work immediately following graduation and the setting in which you see yourself 5 years after graduation (if the same, describe how your duties and caseload might differ with experience). Complete the following chart, describing others with whom you might work at that setting, diagnoses that might be prevalent there, and the skills you have or may need to develop to work at each setting.

	Reasons this setting is a good fit for me	Other providers/ professionals with whom I might work in that setting	Types of patient health conditions commonly seen in this setting	Special skills/ knowledge that might be needed to be successful
Setting where I might work *immediately* after graduation:				
Setting where I might work *5 years after* graduation:				

3

The Preferred Physical Therapist/Physical Therapist Assistant Relationship

CHAPTER OBJECTIVES

After reading this chapter, the reader will be able to:

- Identify key components of the preferred physical therapist/physical therapist assistant (PT/PTA) relationship.
- Compare and contrast PT and PTA educational programs.
- List the responsibilities of each person in an effective PT/PTA team.
- Identify American Physical Therapy Association (APTA) standards, policies, and documents that provide guidance regarding PT and PTA interaction.
- Recognize the PTA's responsibilities in representing physical therapy and the PTA scope of work during interactions with the patient and other members of the health-care team.
- Discuss strategies for resolving conflict in the PT/PTA relationship.

KEY TERMS AND CONCEPTS

- The preferred PT/PTA relationship
- Patient/client management (examination, evaluation, diagnosis, prognosis)
- Plan of care
- Interventions
- Doctor of physical therapy
- Roles and responsibilities
- Patient progression
- PT/PTA communication
- APTA PTA Clinical Problem Solving Algorithm

*C*atherine is an experienced PTA who has worked for many years in an acute care facility. She generally sees most of her patients at bedside, where she frequently interacts with family members and with other members of the health-care team. She attends care conferences and, in consultation with Sasha, her supervising PT, often gives updates to the team regarding the patient's progress

(vignette continues on page 40)

toward goals and discharge. One day, one of the nurses on the unit introduces Catherine as a PT to another new nurse. When Catherine corrects her, the nurse asks about the differences between a PT and a PTA, stating that it appears Catherine does the same tasks as the other therapists on the unit.

QUESTIONS TO CONSIDER

What differences exist between the roles of the PT and PTA? How are these differences demonstrated in the clinical environment? How are these differences explained to patients and other health-care professionals? Is Catherine performing in a role appropriate for a PTA?

At some point, every PTA will likely be asked to explain the difference between the PTA role and that of a PT. This explanation may be given to a patient, a family member, or another health-care provider. PTAs may also have to explain the differences to PTs unfamiliar with the roles PTAs should perform in the clinical setting. It is important that the PTA and PT be able to understand and articulate the differences in their roles and how APTA and regulatory agency policies and legal guidelines affect those roles. This chapter addresses the ways in which the PT and PTA can develop the ability to interact confidently as a true team, developing what is often referred to as **"the preferred PT/PTA relationship."**

Components of the Preferred Relationship

An effective PT/PTA team will achieve its anticipated outcomes most efficiently and effectively if expectations and responsibilities are clear and accepted by both people involved. To make this happen, the PT and PTA need to develop the following:

- Familiarity with each other's educational background
- Understanding of the differences and similarities of each other's role
- Awareness of and trust in each other's skills and knowledge base
- Strategies for effective communication with each other and with others on the health-care team

Role Delineation and Education

As discussed in Chapter 2, the *Guide to Physical Therapist Practice* was developed to help those inside and outside physical therapy practice to understand what PTs do.[1] However, it is also a valuable resource for defining the work of both the PT and

PTA. The *Guide* clearly states that the only providers of physical therapy are the PT and the PTA under the direction and supervision of the PT.[1] The *Guide* describes the various roles of the PT, which include:[1]

- Providing direct patient/client care services in primary, secondary or tertiary (highly specialized) settings to those who have changes in health or function because of injury, illness, disease, or other causes
- Practicing as the principal care provider or in collaboration with other health-care professionals
- Addressing factors or behaviors that put individuals or populations at risk for decreased functional capacity
- Promoting health and wellness by providing preventive services
- Serving as a consultant, educator, administrator, or researcher
- Directing and supervising the physical therapy department and all support personnel, including PTAs and PT aides

FOR REFLECTION

- Most of you have performed some type of observation activity in a physical therapy clinic before beginning your PTA educational program. Did you see these roles exhibited by the PTs you observed? Did you see PTAs in any of these roles?

As a patient/client care provider, the PT is responsible for the elements of **patient/ client management** (see Fig. 3-1). In reviewing these elements, the *Guide* describes four of these areas as being the sole responsibility of the PT:

- **Examination:** obtaining and reviewing the patient's history, performing a systems review (gross assessment of the individual's musculoskeletal, cardiopulmonary, neurological, and integumentary status), and performing various tests and measures to collect meaningful data on the patient's functional abilities.
- **Evaluation:** interpreting and making informed decisions regarding the information and data collected to determine the individual's appropriateness for physical therapy; this information also guides the establishment of the diagnosis, prognosis, and plan of care.
- **Diagnosis:** one or more labels that describe the impact of the activity limitations and participation restrictions identified compared with optimal functional levels, especially in terms of the movement system (see Chapter 1). This diagnosis must also be relative to the tests and measures performed in the examination and within the physical therapist's scope of practice.
- **Prognosis:** a prediction about the amount of improvement anticipated as a result of the physical therapy intervention, as measured by the development of goals and expected outcomes within a given time frame.[1]

These processes culminate in the development of the **plan of care,** which identifies the frequency that the patient/client will be seen (often stated in times per day and/or week), the anticipated duration of the episode of care, and the specific **interventions**

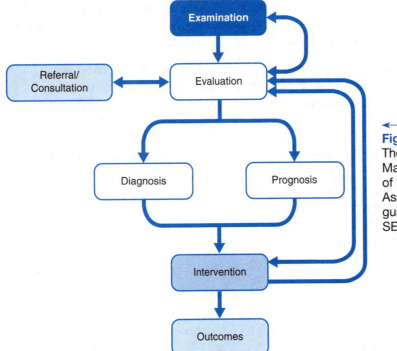

Figure 3-1. The Process of Physical Therapist Patient and Client Management. (Reprinted with permission of the American Physical Therapy Association. Accessed from http://guidetoptpractice.apta.org/content/1/SEC2.body.)

to be performed with that patient/client.[1] *Intervention* is defined in the *Guide* as the delivery of various physical therapy procedures and techniques "to produce changes in the condition that are consistent with the diagnosis and prognosis . . . contingent on the timely monitoring of patient/client response and the progress made toward achieving the anticipated goals and expected outcomes."[1]

Although intervention is the only component of patient/client management to which the PTA directly contributes, it is the one that produces changes in the patient's status and leads to achieving goals and outcomes. Because the application of interventions is the main focus of the work of the entry-level PTA,[2] many PTA programs use some type of competency-based model of skill assessment in which students are expected to demonstrate a minimally acceptable level of skill performance with many different intervention techniques.[3] Because of this, PTA students often perform more laboratory-based practice and testing on their delivery of physical agents, exercise, and other components of intervention than do their PT student counterparts, making the PTA a valuable resource for the PT to use in decision-making regarding the delivery of interventions.

As one would expect, the focus in the PT's educational preparation goes beyond intervention to include the previously identified components of patient/client management. The Commission for Accreditation of Physical Therapy Education (CAPTE) is the accrediting body for both PT and PTA programs, and it differentiates what should be taught to students in each type of curriculum. As part of the entry-level education that culminates in the **doctor of physical therapy** (DPT) degree, today's PT is required to have extensive training in scientific theory and in the application of specific tests and measures to be able to make skilled judgments regarding the causes of patients' functional loss, level of disability, and ability to improve. The PTA's education also has a strong science emphasis but not at the same level as that for the PT. PTA education places less emphasis on the theoretical and evaluative components of physical therapy, but includes exposure to these concepts (e.g., observing a PT perform an examination and listening to the PT explain the evaluative decision-making processes).

The pattern of similar educational topics being covered, but at different depths, is seen again when comparing the nonscience components of PTA and DPT curricula. Ethical decision-making, critical thinking, communication skills, and other traits not unique to physical therapy but essential for success in the profession[4] can be developed in both PTs and PTAs by using feedback informally and formally, using tools such as the "Professional Behaviors for the 21st Century" document (formerly known as the Generic Abilities assessment tool).[5] Whereas the PT student's curriculum includes an emphasis on administration and management that is generally not part of the PTA's educational preparation, leadership development is important for both PTs and PTAs. Chapter 12 discusses the concepts of PTA leadership and professional behavior development in greater detail.

In the clinical setting, the similarities and differences continue. Both PT and PTA students develop and enhance their clinical skills through hundreds of hours of interaction with patients under the supervision of practicing clinicians. Given the shorter length of the PTA associate degree program, the total number of hours in the PTA graduate's clinical education is less than that of the PT graduate. However, both are being educated as generalists and therefore will perform their clinical education in the same types of practice settings, with caseloads representing a wide spectrum of patient diagnoses. In the clinical setting, all PT and PTA programs expect optimal safety and effectiveness in the delivery of physical therapy services, and both programs expect that graduates be able to modify interventions based on the response of the patient. However, in the case of the PTA, the modification of interventions needs to be within the plan of care set up or revised by the PT.[2]

Does that mean that a PTA does not make decisions regarding a patient's status or abilities? Absolutely not. Being able to make decisions regarding the patient's status is expected of PTAs, and the student PTA's ability to do so is developed and assessed in the classroom and during clinical experiences.[2] However, the PTA's decision-making is generally done within a given intervention session on more of a day-to-day basis compared with the PT's level of decision-making, which occurs throughout the entire episode of care to help the patient achieve desired goals. Whether the interventions are provided by the PT or the PTA, the PT retains the ultimate responsibility for their delivery, as oversight and management of the patient rests with the PT.[1] However, when components of care are delivered by the PTA, the PT must be able to rely on the PTA for accurate data collection skills and patient status assessments.

Developing the Preferred PT/PTA Relationship

Upon completing their full rotation of clinical experiences, PTA students often comment that they saw PTAs treated differently and PT/PTA teams interacting differently at each setting. In some settings, students report that PTAs did not have their own daily schedule, did not appear to be encouraged to think independently, and had duties directed to them that appeared most often to be those tasks that the PT simply did not want to perform. In other settings, students noted that the PTAs appeared to be functioning so independently that it was difficult for them to determine who the supervising PT was and that consultation between the PTA and PT appeared to be minimal. Neither of these observations reflects the preferred PT/PTA relationship. In the preferred relationship, the PT/PTA team needs to learn about, understand, and complement each other's skills and aptitudes to allow their partnership to benefit each team partner and the patient. But this is easier said than done, especially given the fast pace and productivity demands of today's health-care environment. The following becomes the challenge to both members of the PT/PTA team:

• Determining what both of them need to do to ensure that they are interacting in the best way possible to meet clinical demands and achieve the best patient outcomes.
• Deciding on the strategies they will use to ensure their partnership works most effectively.

Given that in many settings PTs and PTAs will not be working side by side, a successful team needs to lay the foundation for their working relationship ahead of time. Each team member must develop an awareness of and trust in the other's skill level and knowledge base.[2] They must also be proactive in discussing their expectations concerning the responsibilities of each team member in regard to decision-making, patient progression, and communication. As a result, when the team members are working apart, each will have confidence in the other's ability to perform the designated role appropriately and effectively, maximizing the potential for positive patient outcomes.

FOR REFLECTION
FOR REFLECTION

■ Based on your personality, how do you see yourself wanting to interact with your supervising PT on a daily basis?

Recognizing Strengths and Tendencies

Even though all PTAs go through relatively similar educational programs, there will always be subtle differences in what one program emphasizes versus another. Likewise, each PTA graduate will leave the academic setting with different levels of confidence in performing particular techniques and procedures. Once out in the field, each person continues to develop more advanced skills in certain areas, but has less exposure to others, based on the type of setting and nature of the patients. It is helpful when a PT/PTA team can be familiar with the areas of patient care in which each excels, along with the areas in which each is not so confident. This is especially important for the PT to be able to have a better idea of the amount of supervision that an assigned task might require. If each member of the team recognizes the other's strengths, each is more likely to try to learn from the other and more readily consult with the other. It may be helpful, when appropriate, for a PT/PTA team to attend continuing education opportunities together. This enables them to have first-hand knowledge about each other's familiarity with a particular topic. It may then make it easier for them to incorporate new techniques or intervention approaches into a given patient's plan of care, as both will be approaching it from the same direction.

Along with developing differences in skill sets, clinicians may develop recognizable tendencies regarding how each approaches a given patient. One person may tend to be more aggressive with exercises or might have developed a greater ability to deal with agitated or poorly motivated patients. Even though no one should have to conform to another's personality, it can disrupt the interaction with the patient or other caregivers if the members of the PT/PTA team have very different styles. The PT and PTA need to understand each other's tendencies and recognize when to use those tendencies to the patient's benefit. They should also give each other permission to acknowledge when some tendencies might impede patient progress. One plus of working as a PT/PTA team is that there are two minds looking out for the best interests of the patient.

Finally, PTs and PTAs should recognize that they may have different personality types that can affect the quality of their relationship with others.[6] Differences in behavioral characteristics and learning styles can influence a person's organizational methods, communication preferences, information processing styles, and ways of managing conflict. There is no one "right" personality mix for a PT/PTA team. However, it is important to recognize where variations in personalities might interfere with the team's functioning or when they might be used to enhance patient outcomes. Many tests can be used to formally assess personality and preferred learning style.[6] Physical therapy–specific assessments that can help identify behavioral tendencies include evaluation tools such as the previously mentioned Professional Behaviors assessment and the Clinical Performance Instrument.

How can the PT and PTA learn about each other's strengths with all of the other demands placed on them? It takes effort on the part of both people to ensure that this occurs. The supervisory visits that PTs are required to perform (see Chapter 4) should allow for discussion time and sharing of philosophies. Treating a patient together or working side by side with individual patients gives them the chance to observe each other and their approaches to the patient. Performing chart reviews together, discussing approaches used and decisions made, and then comparing them with patient outcomes can help both team members become more reflective practitioners and aid in their future decision-making. If feasible, it can be extremely helpful for a PTA to sit in on the initial examination and evaluation of a patient who may subsequently be placed in his caseload. That way, the PTA hears firsthand the information that has been shared between the PT and the patient and can witness the approach the PT has taken with the patient. The PTA will then have a better understanding of how the expected goals and outcomes were developed, will be clear on the focus of the interventions to be provided, and can more accurately reinforce any suggestions or instructions initially given to the patient.

Individual Roles and Responsibilities

Both members of the PT/PTA team must clearly understand each other's **roles and responsibilities.** The first task is to ensure that both parties are clear about who is responsible for the various components of patient/client management. Although this may sound obvious, there are many PTs who have had little education about or interaction with PTAs during their careers, and it should not be assumed that every PT is familiar with the PTA's scope of work. Most PTs understand that the PTA cannot perform examinations and evaluations, but they may not be clear on the PTA's ability to progress a patient or on the state regulations regarding PTA direction and supervision. Since the creation of the PTA position, confusion has existed over what PTAs can and cannot do. Robinson et al[7] reported on two surveys in which PTs were asked to identify whether certain tasks were within the APTA's PTA work guidelines. Their results indicated that PTAs were being overutilized in some situations and underutilized in others, with some erroneous perceptions of the PTA's role more pronounced in the later study. A perception that PT students were not being taught enough about the role of the PTA has led CAPTE to write multiple position papers regarding the organization's expectations of how PT/PTA interaction should be addressed in PT and PTA curricula. CAPTE has stated that PT programs must be able to demonstrate that they have sufficiently addressed issues regarding appropriate direction and supervision; those not able to demonstrate this face being cited for noncompliance with CAPTE evaluative criteria.[8] Because of this, recent PT graduates may have a greater familiarity with the role of the PTA than earlier graduates.

It is not just the PT who may be confused about what the PTA can and cannot do. A follow-up study by Robinson et al also found that PTAs disagreed with PTs on about 25% of the tasks in question, with PTAs being less accurate than PTs in determining whether a task was within the PTA's guidelines for performance.[9]

It can be an awkward beginning for a PT/PTA team if one person has to teach the other about the rules and regulations that pertain to the PTA. Often, this can be best handled on a department-wide basis in the form of in-service opportunities (formal or informal educational updates, usually provided on a departmental or facility-wide level). If that does not occur, the PTA should initiate a discussion with the supervising PT about the role of the PTA and the expectations and laws regarding supervision to clarify areas of confusion or disagreement.

Ideally, every PT should be able to articulate what factors will be taken into consideration when deciding what to direct to the PTA. Some PTs may be very conservative in applying these considerations and may not allow the PTA to perform some aspects of care with which the PTA feels very comfortable. Conversely, some PTs may appear to direct tasks indiscriminately. When there is disagreement about which aspects of the patient's care should be directed to the PTA, the PTA needs to remember that the PT retains ultimate responsibility for the patient, including those components of intervention that are performed by the PTA.[10] If the PT and PTA have already discussed the parameters for direction and supervision, the PTA may feel more confident initiating a conversation with the PT about specific issues regarding a given patient. The PTA must also keep in mind the ethical responsibility (and possibly legal duty, depending on state law) to refuse to perform a task that is not within the PTA's scope of work.[11]

The PT and PTA also need to discuss the PTA's ability to make decisions regarding **patient progression.** Patient progression *within the plan of care* is permissible in the PTA's scope of work and part of their educational preparation.[2] In general, within each patient's plan of care, the PTA should be expected to regularly progress intervention intensity (or recognize when it should not be progressed) so that the patient may improve at the fastest rate possible. However, there may be varying levels of complexity involved with these decisions. Many effective PT/PTA teams find it helpful to establish specific parameters for the PTAs to follow within each plan of care and the PTA's scope of work. These parameters will most likely be different for every PT/PTA team, again based on each person's experience and personality. Some PTs would prefer that the PTA consult with them before any change or progression is made, whereas other PTs may have less conservative boundaries for doing so. A less experienced PTA may want to consult with his supervising PT on a regular basis to confirm decisions regarding progression, whereas PTAs with more experience may not feel the need for that reassurance. The PTA must remember that it is *always* necessary to consult with the PT for any change that is outside the patient's plan of care.

FOR REFLECTION

- Return to Chapter 1 and review the four factors that Watts identified for PTs to consider in deciding what tasks to direct to a PTA. How might a PT's overall experience or familiarity with the role of the PTA affect understanding of PTAs and patient progression?

Communication Styles and Strategies: Planning for Interaction

Obviously, to learn about each other's roles, the PT and PTA must engage in some form of **communication.** However, just as people have different personalities, they also have different communication styles and preferences. It is extremely important for an effective PT/PTA team to establish protocols for how the two people can best communicate with each other. Each person first needs to self-identify areas of strength, weakness, and preference in communicating with others. For example, some people are more assertive whereas others are more reserved; some need more processing time than others who can quickly "think on their feet," and some retain written information better than spoken words. Discussing one's preferred style of communicating, giving feedback, and dealing with conflict are all helpful because the team can then recognize areas of similarity and difference. This discussion is of particular importance if the team members have different cultural backgrounds, as one's culture can have a significant impact on communication preferences and how one interprets communication from others.[12] Observing each other during care conferences or interactions with family members can further help each team member be more familiar with the other's style.

FOR REFLECTION

FOR REFLECTION

- Describe your communication style.

Once communication styles are established, the PT/PTA team may then establish the processes to be used for discussion and collaboration regarding patient care. The APTA states in its position on direction and supervision that "there must be regularly scheduled and documented conferences with the physical therapist assistant regarding patients/clients, the frequency of which is determined by the needs of the patient/client and the needs of the physical therapist assistant."[9] The decision on how and when to best hold these meetings may be determined in part by the physical proximity of supervision regularly provided by the PT. Those PT/PTA teams who work in close physical contact may be able to consult with each other throughout the course of the day. However, when the supervising PT is not in the building at all times, or if the PT and PTA work in different parts of a building, it may be more effective for the team to set regular meeting times to discuss patients. The PT/PTA team must always follow the laws regarding proximity of supervision for their state, but for most effective PT/PTA teams, those laws are a minimum required level of supervision and not the preferred amount of interaction. Each member of the PT/PTA team needs to recognize that each may have additional responsibilities in a given day beyond direct patient care. These responsibilities may include participation in meetings with families, other health-care disciplines, or facility committees; attending continuing education or training in-service sessions; billing and scheduling duties; and other managerial or administrative tasks. All of these, as well as differences in scheduled work hours (for example, if one leaves earlier than the other or differences in meal breaks), can affect when and how interaction occurs.

Regular meetings are important, but sometimes communication must take place on the spur of the moment. For many PTAs, especially new ones, knowing when to consult with the supervising PT can be a challenge. One tool that can be extremely helpful is the **APTA PTA Clinical Problem Solving Algorithm** (Fig. 3-2). Designed to supplement the regularly scheduled ongoing meetings that occur between the PT and the PTA, the algorithm was created to assist the PTA in decision-making while delivering interventions.[13] It can also serve to remind the PT to provide appropriate direction to the PTA and opportunities for ongoing communication. PTAs must remember that they need to be proactive in finding answers to questions and clarifying information. PTs are rarely able to anticipate every question that the PTA might have. If the directions and parameters for progression are not clear, the PTA has the responsibility to seek out further information; the algorithm in Figure 3-2 has the potential of empowering PTAs to feel more comfortable in doing so. Additional APTA algorithms for PTs to use in decision-making related to direction and supervision are presented in Chapter 4.

Problem Solving Algorithm Utilized by PTAs in Patient/Client Intervention

This algorithm, developed by APTA's Departments of Education, Accreditation, and Practice, is intended to reflect current policies and positions on the problem solving processes utilized by physical therapist assistants in the provision of selected interventions. The controlling assumptions are essential to understanding and applying this algorithm. (This document can be found in *A Normative Model of Physical Therapist Assistant Education: Version 2007.*)

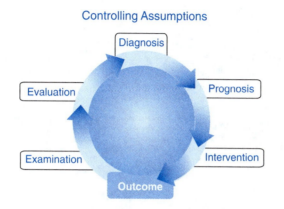

- The physical therapist integrates the five elements of patient/client management – examination, evaluation, diagnosis, prognosis, and intervention – in a manner designed to optimize outcomes. Responsibility for completion of the examination, evaluation, diagnosis, and prognosis is borne solely by the physical therapist. The physical therapist's plan of care may involve the physical therapist assistant to assist with selected interventions. This algorithm represents the decision making of the physical therapist assistant within the intervention element.

- The physical therapist will direct and supervise the physical therapist assistant consistent with APTA House of Delegates positions, including Direction and Supervision of the Physical Therapist Assistant (HOD P06-05-18-26); APTA core documents, including Standards of Ethical Conduct for the PTA; and federal and state legal practice standards; and institutional regulations.

- All selected interventions are directed and supervised by the physical therapist. Additionally, the physical therapist remains responsible for the physical therapy services provided when the physical therapist's plan of care involves the physical therapist assistant to assist with selected interventions.

- Selected intervention(s) includes the procedural intervention, associated data collection, and communication, including written documentation associated with the safe, effective, and efficient completion of the task.

- The algorithm may represent the thought processes involved in a patient/client interaction or episode of care. Entry into the algorithm will depend on the point at which the physical therapist assistant is directed by the physical therapist to provide selected interventions.

- Communication between the physical therapist and physical therapist assistant regarding patient/client care is ongoing. The algorithm does not intend to imply a limitation or restriction on communication between the physical therapist and physical therapist assistant.

Figure 3-2. APTA PTA Clinical Problem Solving Algorithm. (Reprinted with permission of the American Physical Therapy Association. Accessed from http://www.apta.org/PTA/PatientCare/.)   *Continued*

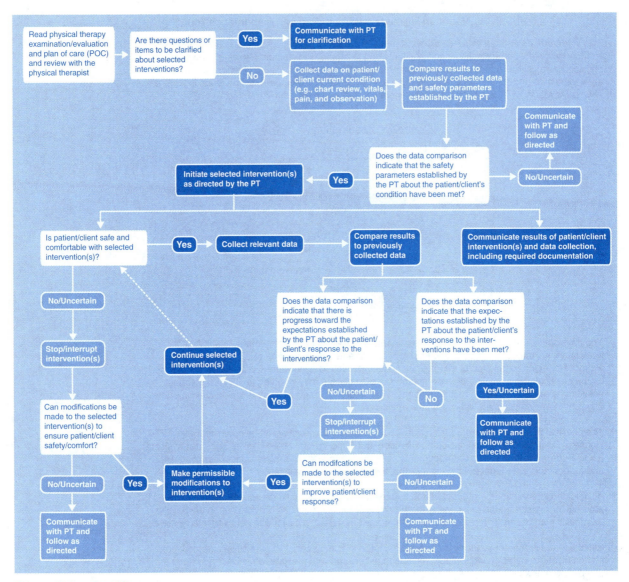

Figure 3-2.—cont'd

Parameters for Communication With Others

Patients, their families, and other caregivers will have questions throughout the course of a patient's episode of care, and it is important for the PT/PTA team to anticipate these and establish, as best they can, which questions the PTA should answer and which should be directed to the PT. The same is true of questions from other members of the health-care team, the facility's administration, or outside entities such as third-party payers. In general, questions containing an evaluative component, such as when a patient will be ready for discharge to a lesser level of care, should always be referred to the PT. However, it would most likely be appropriate for a PTA to report on the patient's current status regarding progress toward the goals established by the PT or to comment on identified barriers toward discharge. In addition, a PTA should be able to:

- Answer questions regarding the rationale for performing an exercise or technique or using a physical agent during an intervention session
- Share knowledge regarding a patient diagnosis
- Discuss relevant factual information from clinical experience

The PTA should make sure that the person with whom he is speaking knows that he is speaking from the perspective of a PTA and that further clarification from the PT might be warranted. The PTA should let the other person know that he will update the PT regarding the questions asked so that the PT has the opportunity to provide a more in-depth assessment or more detailed information, as appropriate. A PTA should never attempt to answer a question that is outside his scope of work and should be comfortable in stating when he does not know or cannot answer a question. It is better to err on the side of referring to or consulting with the PT than to overstep the PTA's scope of work. The individual asking the question will be best served if the PTA takes responsibility for following through to find the answer or pass the question on to someone who is in a more appropriate position to provide the answer.

Resolving Conflict

Misunderstanding or tension between members of the PT/PTA team can often be traced back to a difference in expectations. When miscommunication happens, team members must work together to identify where the breakdown occurred to prevent it from happening again. Use of the previously mentioned APTA algorithms can help each member of the team identify where alternative communication, consultation, decision-making, or action should have occurred.[13]

It is not always necessary, or even helpful, to try to identify who was "wrong" in a given scenario. If both members of the partnership have previously acknowledged their joint responsibility toward making the team work effectively, then it is not necessary to place blame, only to learn from the situation and make sure that any miscommunication or misunderstanding is corrected. It may be advantageous to review any preestablished protocols or responsibilities to clarify roles. If, for some reason, these parameters were not established initially, then the team should take the responsibility for doing so immediately. If one or both members of the team are resistant, a departmental supervisor may take the role of mediator. It is the PT's responsibility to direct and supervise appropriately, and, if this is not occurring, the PTA has no other choice but to bring in someone else to help remediate the situation.

Specific techniques to facilitate effective communication with patients are addressed in Chapter 6.

FOR REFLECTION

- How do you respond to conflict? How could that affect how you interact with your PT/PTA team partner in times of stress or disagreement?

Working With Multiple Therapists

Depending on state law, the staffing at a given site, and the demands placed on the staff at that site, it is possible that a PTA may be supervised by more than one PT during the course of a workweek or even on a given day. The challenges of working as a successful team are magnified when multiple supervising PTs are involved. It is not unusual for the PTA taking direction from multiple PTs to receive conflicting messages on how to approach a given patient or on each PT's parameters for progression within the plan of care. Proactive communication is essential in this kind of situation. Some PTAs find that it is helpful to keep some type of journal to keep track of the PT responsible for each patient, along with a record of that PT's preferences and parameters for progression. Observing each PT's interactions with patients can be very useful for the PTA to ensure each approach to a given patient. It is like being a "chameleon," adapting one's style to that of each PT with whom one works, as a way of anticipating and diffusing potential problems.[14]

Some patients in the PTA's caseload may have had their initial examination and evaluations performed by PTs within the facility who do not continue as the supervising PT for that patient. This can occur, for example, when a patient is initially seen by a weekend-only PT and is transferred to a different PT's caseload for intervention sessions during the week. In this type of situation, especially in larger departments, it may be challenging for the PTA to know who is responsible for that patient's care or to whom the PTA should go for consultation in case of questions or concerns. The APTA has established a position that encourages the development of protocols within a department to ensure appropriate establishment of the "physical therapist of record" and "hand-off" communication procedures, which can help PTAs be clear on who is responsible for each patient and to whom they should go when questions arise.[15]

SUMMARY

The successful PT/PTA team is one in which both members are able to describe their own and their partner's role in the delivery of physical therapy services. They must demonstrate an awareness of and respect for each other's educational background and must trust in each other's skills. This can be encouraged by observing each other's work with patients and by sharing reflections regarding one's own abilities with the other. The successful PT/PTA team will develop consistent approaches for ensuring appropriate communication with each other, with others in the health-care team, and with patients and their families. Use of tools such as the APTA PTA Clinical Problem Solving Algorithm can facilitate improved communication. By developing proactive protocols and strategies for interaction, the PT/PTA team will be able to work most efficiently, combining the strengths of their individual roles to maximize patient outcomes.

REFERENCES

1. American Physical Therapy Association. *Guide to Physical Therapist Practice 3.0.* Alexandria, VA: American Physical Therapy Association. http://guidetoptpractice.apta.org/. Updated 2014. Accessed July 6, 2015.

2. American Physical Therapy Association. *A Normative Model of Physical Therapist Assistant Education: Version 2007.* Alexandria, VA: American Physical Therapy Association; 2007.

3. US Department of Education, National Post-Secondary Educational Cooperative. Defining and assessing learning: exploring competency-based initiatives. 2002.

4. May WW, Morgan BJ, Lemke JC, Karst GM, Stone HL. Model for ability-based assessment in physical therapy education. *J Phys Ther Educ.* 1995;9(1):3-6.

5. May W, Kontney L, Iglarsh Z. Professional behaviors for the 21st century 2009-2010. http://www.marquette.edu/physical-therapy/documents/ProfessionalBehaviors.pdf. Accessed August 13, 2015.

6. Coyne C. Understanding PT, PTA, and patient personality types. *PT Magazine.* 2004;12(4).

7. Robinson AJ, McCall M, DePalma MT, et al. Physical therapists' perceptions of the roles of the physical therapist assistant. *Phys Ther.* 1994;74(6):571-582.

8. Commission on Accreditation in Physical Therapy Education. Expectations for the education of physical therapists and physical therapist assistants regarding direction and supervision. 2013:18-19.

9. Robinson AJ, DePalma MT, McCall M. Physical therapist assistants' perceptions of the documented roles of the physical therapist assistant. *Phys Ther.* 1995;75(12):1054-1064.

10. American Physical Therapy Association. Direction and supervision of the physical therapist assistant (HOD P06-05-18-26). http://www.apta.org/uploadedFiles/APTAorg/About_Us/Policies/Practice/DirectionSupervisionPTA.pdf. Updated 2012. Accessed August 13, 2015.

11. American Physical Therapy Association. Standards of ethical conduct for the physical therapist assistant. http://www.apta.org/uploadedFiles/APTAorg/About_Us/Policies/Ethics/StandardsEthicalConductPTA.pdf. Updated 2015. Accessed August 13, 2015.

12. Lattanzi JB, Purnell, LD. *Developing Cultural Competence in Physical Therapy Practice.* Philadelphia, PA: FA Davis; 2006:417.

13. American Physical Therapy Association. PTA Clinical Problem Solving Algorithm. http://www.apta.org/PTA/PatientCare/. Updated 2007. Accessed August 13, 2015.

14. Solberg JJ. Personal communication. May 1, 2009.

15. American Physical Therapy Association. Physical therapist of record and "hand off" communication (HOD P06-08-16-16). http://www.apta.org/uploadedFiles/APTAorg/About_Us/Policies/Practice/RecordHandOffCommunication.pdf. Updated 2012. Accessed August 13, 2015.

Name _____

REVIEW

1. Identify four key components of an effective PT/PTA team, and explain why they are important in creating the preferred PT/PTA relationship.

   _____

   _____

   _____

   _____

   _____

2. List three similarities and three differences in the educational processes of PTs and PTAs.

   _____

   _____

   _____

3. Explain why it is important for a PT/PTA team to have trust in each other's abilities.

   _____

   _____

   _____

   _____

4. Whose responsibility is it to ensure that all directions and parameters for patient progression have been clarified? Explain your answer.

   _____

   _____

   _____

   _____

(questions continue on page 56)

Application

1. Catherine, the PTA described at the beginning of this chapter, is working with a patient who asks some questions regarding how much improvement he should expect to make. Catherine refers him to Sasha, the supervising PT, saying, "I'm a PTA. I can't answer questions about prognosis." Do you agree with the way Catherine answered the patient's question? Why or why not? If not, what would you do differently?

   _____

   _____

   _____

   _____

2. The patient's wife says, "I know someone who is a PTA. She says that a PTA can do everything a PT can do except evaluations, right?" How would you respond?

   _____

   _____

   _____

   _____

3. As a newly graduated PTA, you will be working with at least one PT. Identify at least one trait that you will need to develop between now and then to contribute more positively to the PT/PTA team relationship. Describe what you might do to help develop that trait.

   _____

   _____

   _____

   _____

4

Regulatory Requirements for Direction and Supervision of the Physical Therapist Assistant

CHAPTER OBJECTIVES

After reading this chapter, the reader will be able to:

- Identify the various organizations and regulatory bodies that influence the scope of work of the physical therapist assistant (PTA).
- Differentiate between various types of state regulations for PTAs.
- Give examples of different types of regulations pertaining to PTAs that might appear within a state's practice act.
- Describe how the regulatory requirements for PTAs may vary from state to state (or within practice settings).
- Discuss the implications for not abiding by American Physical Therapy Association (APTA) viewpoints.
- Compare and contrast the levels of supervision defined by the APTA.
- Describe typical licensure requirements for PTAs.
- Discuss the regulatory requirements that must be considered to provide appropriate supervision of physical therapy students.

KEY TERMS AND CONCEPTS

- Direction
- Supervision
- Statutes
- Practice act
- Rules
- Federation of State Boards of Physical Therapy (FSBPT)
- Supervisory visit
- Supervision ratio
- APTA viewpoints: guidelines, positions, standards
- APTA levels of supervision: general, direct, direct personal
- APTA PTA Direction Algorithm and APTA PTA Supervision Algorithm
- National Physical Therapy Examination (NPTE)
- Jurisprudence examination

Rashan *is a recent graduate of a PTA program located in a neighboring state. He has taken a position in a growing rehabilitation department within a skilled nursing facility. On his first day, he learns that he will be paired up with Samira, a physical therapist (PT) who has worked at the facility for 2 years. On the first day, Samira tells Rashan that their department has never had a PTA working in it and asks him whether he is familiar with the rules and regulations that pertain to the PTA. Rashan tells her about the rules he followed during his clinical training but then remembers that those clinicals were not performed in the state where he is currently working. He hesitates and says, "I'm not sure if I do, but I think I know where I can find them."*

QUESTIONS TO CONSIDER

Are the rules that apply to PTA supervision consistent from state to state? What resources can Rashan use to learn about the regulations? Are there other factors beyond state regulations that will affect what tasks Samira directs Rashan to perform? Do student PTAs follow the same regulations as do PTA graduates?

According to the *Guide to Physical Therapist Practice,* "direction and supervision are essential to the provision of high-quality physical therapy."[1] Earlier chapters discussed the decision-making process that needs to occur when a PT chooses to direct a PTA to perform certain components of a patient's intervention and to ensure those components are performed appropriately. This chapter focuses on the regulatory agency and professional association guidelines that influence how **direction** (assigning portions of the intervention or other tasks to the PTA) and **supervision** (ensuring the PTA performs her assigned duties properly) should be performed by the PT. The PT is responsible for directing and supervising the PTA, but both the PT and the PTA must understand the legal and regulatory requirements to ensure this is done correctly. Every PTA must ensure she is receiving appropriate supervision and is performing only the tasks for which she is qualified. She must be knowledgeable regarding state laws, APTA policies, and third-party payer guidelines that pertain to the PTA. She must be able to recognize discrepancies between these regulations and what is being delegated or how supervision is being provided; if this occurs, she must be able to bring these issues to the attention of the supervising PT proactively and respectfully.

The PTA must always function "under the direction and supervision of a physical therapist."[2] A PTA cannot work in isolation without a supervising PT. However, depending on the state, the setting, and the particular PTs and PTAs involved, the amount of supervision provided and the types of interventions that the PTA is directed to perform may vary. A PT supervising two PTAs may choose to have one PTA perform a given intervention but not the other. Likewise, she may choose to supervise the two PTAs at two different levels within the guidelines allowable by law. These choices will depend on a number of factors, including the two PTAs' levels of experience, the complexity of the tasks involved, and the risk to the patient if something adverse happens. Similarly, one PTA may need more supervision than another, even more than is required by law, because she is inexperienced with a certain technique or patient diagnosis or because she has questions on how to proceed with delivery or progression of the patient's interventions within the plan of care. Discussions between the members of a PT/PTA team concerning expectations for supervision, patient progression, and intrateam/interteam communication can be helpful in establishing parameters for interaction.

As a PTA becomes more experienced, she typically becomes more confident in her ability to work independently with patients. Similarly, the supervising PT typically develops more confidence and trust in the PTA's abilities to perform without constant oversight and direction. As this occurs, it is even more important to remember the requirements for direction and supervision that pertain to the PT/PTA team, especially as they are written in law, because the law represents a minimum level of regulation that must be maintained, no matter how strong the PTA's abilities.

State Regulation: Practice Acts

Numerous federal laws affect the provision of physical therapy, but the day-to-day practice of physical therapy is regulated at the state level. Each state has its own set of legal **statutes** that delineate the parameters under which physical therapy services can be delivered. These statutory laws are commonly referred to as a state's physical therapy **practice act.** The statutes within a given practice act are written and passed by that state's legislature. Practice acts are developed to protect the public and ensure the competence of those providing the services.[3] However, the statutes also delineate the scope of practice of a given profession. In some cases, they may have very specific parameters, but in others the wording may be more vague, sometimes to avoid being overly restrictive. Statutes may be accompanied by sets of administrative **rules,** which give further clarity to the statements in the statutes.[4] The rules are generally written by the state governing body that oversees the actions of the given profession. This could be a state physical therapy board, a medical board, or a general licensing board.[5]

Because of the challenges involved with maintaining consistency in the profession when laws vary from state to state, a national organization was formed in 1986 to help state boards work together to promote the highest level of public safety. Currently, the state boards of all 50 states and those overseeing the District of Columbia, Puerto Rico, and the U.S. Virgin Islands are members of the **Federation of State Boards of Physical Therapy (FSBPT).**[6] The FSBPT has developed a Model Practice Act, considered to be a "preeminent standard" for states to follow as they attempt to update and clarify their practice acts through legislative change. It provides examples of language to use and content to include in an attempt to make practice acts more uniform from state to state.[7] As with any attempt to modify existing laws, making changes to a practice act can be a lengthy, challenging process. Information about how various types of laws are created is provided in Chapter 10.

In accordance with the Model Practice Act, most state physical therapy practice acts identify, define, or describe the following:

- The terms "physical therapy," "physical therapist," "physical therapist assistant," and other terms associated with the profession, including who can use the terms/titles (also known as "title protection")[3]
- The types of services that PTs (and PTAs) are and are not allowed to provide
- The circumstances under which direct access to physical therapy services is allowed (see Chapter 1)
- The type of licensure or other regulation required for PTs and PTAs
- The educational and national examination requirements for obtaining and maintaining licensure or certification
- The state organization (i.e., PT board, medical board) responsible for overseeing the activities of the licensees
- The providers from whom PTs may accept referrals (physicians, podiatrists, nurse practitioners, physician assistants, and dentists, among others)
- The utilization of the PTA and others who may be connected to the delivery of physical therapy services (PT aides, athletic trainers, students, etc.), including supervision requirements and restrictions to what tasks can be directed to them

The specifics of each of these categories vary from state to state. In addition, practice acts may include other content not mentioned here. All PTs and PTAs need to be familiar with the physical therapy practice act of the state in which they live or are employed. State statutes are public records, and online versions of state statutes and rules are generally easily accessible through a state legislature website or that of the state regulating board or APTA chapter. In addition, the FSBPT website has a page that contains links to every state's licensing board and practice act.[6]

FOR REFLECTION

- Find a copy of your state's physical therapy practice act. Briefly review it to see whether it addresses all the topics noted in the previous section. What is your overall impression of its clarity and how well it addresses the utilization of the PTA?

Variations in PTA Regulation

As of 2015, all 50 states and the District of Columbia regulate physical therapist assistants. However, there are significant variations from state to state in the type of regulation required for PTAs, including the requirements for initial and continuing licensure, the level of physical supervision required (including requirements for supervisory visits and documentation of supervision), PT/PTA supervision ratios, whether PTAs can supervise PT aides, and limitations concerning what duties can be delegated. These topics are addressed individually in the following sections to identify the most common areas in which potential differences might occur.

Licensure

The term "licensure" is often used generically to refer to the legal credential that must be obtained to work as a PTA, but three different levels of regulation can potentially be used, as determined by a given state:[3]

- *Registration:* Generally thought of as least restrictive, registration is used when the risk to the public is generally low. Usually, there is no requirement for specific training or education. It might only consist of providing the state with one's name and address.
- *Certification:* Used for a higher level of regulation, certification usually requires some type of specific education and passing an examination as a way of demonstrating a minimum level of competence.
- *Licensure:* This highest level of oversight is used when the risk to the public is thought to be greatest. In addition to the above, those who are licensed generally are subject to discipline by a state board if they fail to meet regulatory standards.

Currently, the FSBPT includes language referring both to certification and licensure in the Model Practice Act.[7] Information on how to obtain and maintain licensure (or other type of credential, as required) is provided in Chapter 14.

FOR REFLECTION

- Look up your state's physical therapy practice act. What is the level of regulation required for PTAs in your state? Do you think this is an appropriate level of oversight?

Physical Supervision

The practice act should describe the type of supervision exercised by the PT while the PTA is working. Some states may require the PT to be in the same building, whereas others may allow the PT to work at a different location as long as she is easily reachable by some form of telecommunication (phone, pager, computer, etc.). A practice act may also describe some period of face-to-face interaction of the PT and PTA, commonly referred to as a **supervisory visit.** Specific parameters of this visit may include how often it needs to occur, either related to an actual time frame (i.e., once per week, every 30 days) or related to the frequency of patient intervention sessions (i.e., every sixth visit), what needs to occur at the visit (observation, communication, care plan review, etc.), and what needs to be documented.

PT/PTA Supervision Ratios

Many practice acts have restrictions on the number of PTAs that a PT can supervise at any given time. This is referred to as a **supervision ratio.** Some states do not address this issue in their practice acts, and some states' ratio guidelines apply beyond supervision of PTAs to include aides, students, or other types of support personnel.[6]

Limitations to Intervention Delivery

Practice acts may restrict what the PTA is allowed to perform in the clinic, either by listing that which cannot be done by anyone other than the PT or by identifying responsibilities that the PT cannot delegate to others. For the most part, these are uniformly in line with the PTA's scope of work and educational background (e.g., not being able to perform initial examinations or developing the plan of care), but one state may prohibit a PTA from performing interventions or duties that are allowable in another. For example, some states allow PTAs to be responsible for supervising PT aides in the clinical setting but other states do not.[6]

Others

Other laws on the state and federal level apply to PTs and PTAs, although they are not specific to the profession itself. Many of these laws are covered in Chapter 10.

APTA Policies Regarding Direction and Supervision

In addition to state statutes, the positions of the APTA need to be considered by the PT as she makes decisions regarding how to direct and supervise the PTA. The APTA has many positions and documents that describe the differences in the responsibilities of the PT versus the PTA. These positions are not legally binding but they do represent "best practice" as defined by the APTA, and not following recommended practice guidelines could be used against a practitioner should a lawsuit be filed.[4] Although some state regulations may coincide with APTA guidelines, many do not, with some states' requirements being more restrictive than others on the utilization of the PTA. In many cases, a state's practice act may be silent on a particular practice issue, meaning that it does not address the topic. In such cases, APTA standards can be used. The PTA must remember that her scope of work must always be determined first by her state's practice act and then refined within the guidelines laid out by the APTA.

APTA Viewpoints

Policies that are debated and voted on by the House of Delegates are classified into three categories, and each has a different level of expectation for compliance. **Guidelines** are the least binding, as they are considered a "statement of advice," whereas **positions** are considered to be "a firmly held association stance or point of view" that members are expected to follow. **Standards** have the highest level of expectation for compliance, because they are "a binding statement used to judge quality of action or activity" and often pertain to "right or wrong" conduct, such as that found in the Code of Ethics.[8] Examples of APTA standards include core documents such as the "Standards of Ethical Conduct for the Physical Therapist Assistant" (see Chapter 5). Members who are found to have violated a standard such as this could face being barred from future APTA membership.[4] "Policies" and "procedures" are also terms used to differentiate types of APTA stances; these generally refer to administrative responsibilities.[8]

The APTA has a very detailed position statement, "Direction and Supervision of the PTA," that describes its expectations and specifies those duties for which the PT should have sole responsibility.[2] Again, these may be stated differently from what is contained in a state's practice act and may include or exclude duties singled out by a given state.

Direction and Supervision of the Physical Therapist Assistant (HOD P06-05-18-26)

Physical therapists have a responsibility to deliver services in ways that protect the public safety and maximize the availability of their services. They do this through direct delivery of services in conjunction with responsible utilization of physical therapist assistants who assist with selected components of intervention. The physical therapist assistant is the only individual permitted to assist a physical therapist in selected interventions under the direction and supervision of a physical therapist.

Direction and supervision are essential in the provision of quality physical therapy services. The degree of direction and supervision necessary for assuring quality physical therapy services is dependent upon many factors, including the education, experiences, and responsibilities of the parties involved, as well as the organizational structure in which the physical therapy services are provided.

Regardless of the setting in which the physical therapy service is provided, the following responsibilities must be borne solely by the physical therapist:
1. Interpretation of referrals when available.
2. Initial examination, evaluation, diagnosis, and prognosis.
3. Development or modification of a plan of care that is based on the initial examination or reexamination and that includes the physical therapy goals and outcomes.
4. Determination of when the expertise and decision-making capability of the physical therapist requires the physical therapist to personally render physical therapy interventions and when it may be appropriate to utilize the physical therapist assistant. A physical therapist shall determine the most appropriate

(box continues on page 64)

Direction and Supervision of the Physical Therapist Assistant (HOD P06-05-18-26) (continued)

utilization of the physical therapist assistant that provides for the delivery of service that is safe, effective, and efficient.

5. Reexamination of the patient/client in light of their goals, and revision of the plan of care when indicated.
6. Establishment of the discharge plan and documentation of discharge summary/ status.
7. Oversight of all documentation for services rendered to each patient/client.

The physical therapist remains responsible for the physical therapy services provided when the physical therapist's plan of care involves the physical therapist assistant to assist with selected interventions. Regardless of the setting in which the service is provided, the determination to utilize physical therapist assistants for selected interventions requires the education, expertise, and professional judgment of a physical therapist as described by the *Standards of Practice, Guide to Professional Conduct, and Code of Ethics.*

In determining the appropriate extent of assistance from the physical therapist assistant (PTA), the physical therapist considers:

- The PTA's education, training, experience, and skill level.
- Patient/client criticality, acuity, stability, and complexity.
- The predictability of the consequences.
- The setting in which the care is being delivered.
- Federal and state statutes.
- Liability and risk management concerns
- The mission of physical therapy services for the setting.
- The needed frequency of reexamination
- Physical Therapist Assistant

Definition

The physical therapist assistant is a technically educated health care provider who assists the physical therapist in the provision of physical therapy. The physical therapist assistant is a graduate of a physical therapist assistant associate degree program accredited by the Commission on Accreditation in Physical Therapy Education (CAPTE).

Utilization

The physical therapist is directly responsible for the actions of the physical therapist assistant related to patient/client management. The physical therapist assistant may perform selected physical therapy interventions under the direction and at least general supervision of the physical therapist. In general supervision, the physical therapist is not required to be on-site for direction and supervision, but must be available at least by telecommunications. The ability of the physical therapist assistant to perform the selected interventions as directed shall be assessed on an ongoing basis by the supervising physical therapist. The physical therapist assistant makes modifications to selected interventions either to progress the patient/client as directed by the physical therapist or to ensure patient/client safety and comfort.

Direction and Supervision of the Physical Therapist Assistant (HOD P06-05-18-26) (continued)

The physical therapist assistant must work under the direction and at least general supervision of the physical therapist. In all practice settings, the performance of selected interventions by the physical therapist assistant must be consistent with safe and legal physical therapist practice, and shall be predicated on the following factors: complexity and acuity of the patient's/client's needs; proximity and accessibility to the physical therapist; supervision available in the event of emergencies or critical events; and type of setting in which the service is provided.

When supervising the physical therapist assistant in any off-site setting, the following requirements must be observed:

1. A physical therapist must be accessible by telecommunications to the physical therapist assistant at all times while the physical therapist assistant is treating patients/clients.
2. There must be regularly scheduled and documented conferences with the physical therapist assistant regarding patients/clients, the frequency of which is determined by the needs of the patient/client and the needs of the physical therapist assistant.
3. In those situations in which a physical therapist assistant is involved in the care of a patient/client, a supervisory visit by the physical therapist will be made:
   a. Upon the physical therapist assistant's request for a reexamination, when a change in the plan of care is needed, prior to any planned discharge, and in response to a change in the patient's/client's medical status.
   b. At least once a month, or at a higher frequency when established by the physical therapist, in accordance with the needs of the patient/client.
   c. A supervisory visit should include:
      i. An on-site reexamination of the patient/client.
      ii. On-site review of the plan of care with appropriate revision or termination.
      iii. Evaluation of need and recommendation for utilization of outside resources.

Reprinted with permission of the American Physical Therapy Association. Found at http://www.apta.org/Policies/. Accessed August 13, 2015.

APTA Levels of Supervision

As previously mentioned, many state practice acts specify the type of supervision needed for PTAs (and other supportive personnel). However, many different terms are used to refer to that supervision. The APTA has developed specific hierarchical definitions for three types of supervision that are used with support personnel.[9] If a PTA's state practice act refers to one of these types of supervision, she must determine whether it is being defined in the same way that the APTA has defined it.

General supervision is the least restrictive of the three and is the level of supervision that the APTA believes should be used in supervising the PTA (see

"Direction and Supervision of the Physical Therapist Assistant"). At this level, the PT is not required to be in the same building as the PTA while the PTA is delivering interventions.[2] The next level, **direct supervision,** requires the on-site presence of the PT and daily interaction between the supervising PT and each patient/client being seen by the supervisee. The APTA recommends this level of supervision for PT and PTA students.[10,11] The final level of supervision, **direct personal supervision,** requires the PT (or, where allowed by state law, a PTA) not only to be physically present but also to continually direct and supervise the person who is performing the tasks. The APTA states that this level of supervision should be maintained when PTs and PTAs use the assistance of PT aides.[12]

Levels of Supervision (HOD P06-00-15-26)

The American Physical Therapy Association recognizes the following levels of supervision:

General Supervision: The physical therapist is not required to be on site for direction and supervision, but must be available at least by telecommunications.

Direct Supervision: The physical therapist is physically present and immediately available for direction and supervision. The physical therapist will have direct contact with the patient/client during each visit that is defined in the *Guide to Physical Therapist Practice* as all encounters with a patient/client in a 24-hour period. Telecommunications does not meet the requirement of direct supervision.

Direct Personal Supervision: The physical therapist or, where allowable by law, the physical therapist assistant is physically present and immediately available to direct and supervise tasks that are related to patient/client management. The direction and supervision is continuous throughout the time these tasks are performed. Telecommunications does not meet the requirement of direct personal supervision.

APTA Algorithms for Direction and Supervision

In addition to its formal stances that direct the work of the PTA, the APTA has developed documents and other resources to help PTs and PTAs understand the complexities of direction and supervision. The Clinical Problem Solving Algorithm for PTAs (Chapter 3) is an example of one such item. The **APTA PTA Direction Algorithm** (Fig. 4-1) and the **APTA PTA Supervision Algorithm** (Fig. 4-2) are additional guides to help the PT decide which interventions are appropriate for the PTA to perform, when it is appropriate to direct the PTA to perform those interventions, and the various factors that might determine the appropriate amount of supervision required after the interventions have been directed to the PTA.[13] Like the PTA's algorithm, these newer algorithms apply APTA standards and positions in a step-by-step guide to the decisions and choices that the supervising PT makes when choosing to utilize the PTA in the delivery of physical therapy interventions.

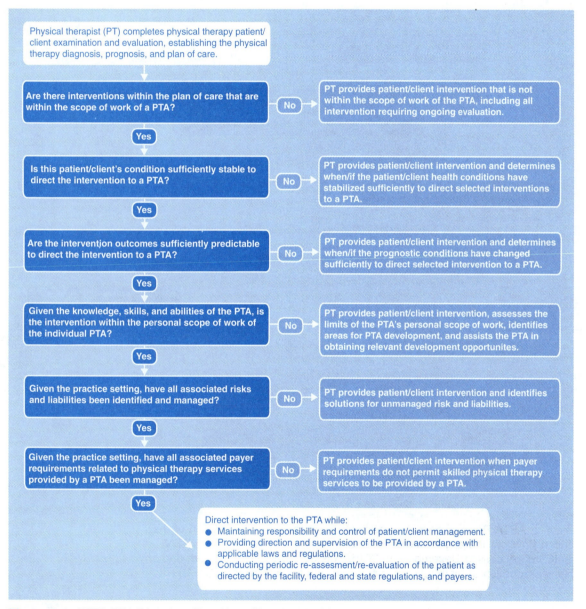

Figure 4-1. APTA PTA Direction Algorithm. (Reprinted with permission of the American Physical Therapy Association. Located at http://www.apta.org/PTA/ PatientCare/. Accessed December 29, 2015. This material is copyrighted, and any further reproduction or distribution requires written permission from APTA.)

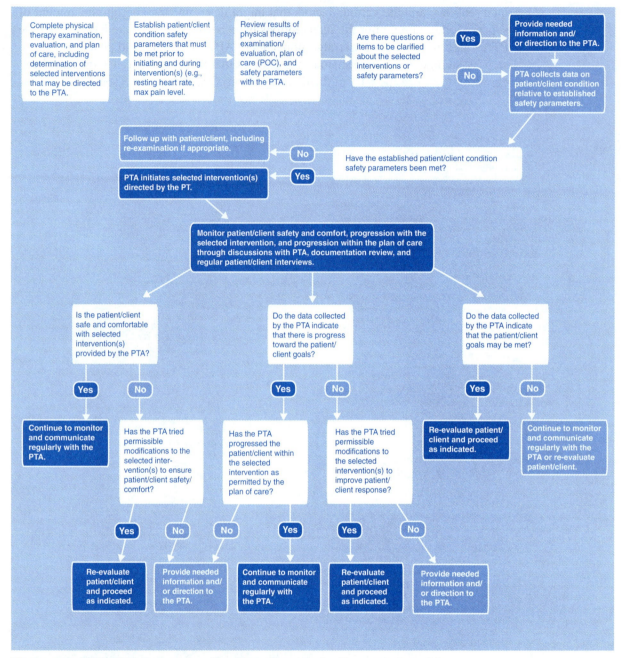

Figure 4-2. APTA PTA Supervision Algorithm. (Reprinted with permission of the American Physical Therapy Association. Located at http://www.apta.org/PTA/PatientCare/. Accessed December 29, 2015. This material is copyrighted, and any further reproduction or distribution requires written permission from APTA.)

These diagrams and many other resources can be found by following the PTA link on the APTA's website (www.apta.org/PTA). Many of the APTA positions that have implications for the PTA are also posted on the APTA's PTA web page.[14]

Third-Party Payer Regulation

Finally, the requirements of third-party payers must be taken into consideration, as they can affect the PTA's ability to participate in certain aspects of patient care delivery and the documentation required regarding those services. Even though it may be legal for a PTA to perform a certain task or to work under a certain level of supervision, if the PTA utilization does not match the requirements set by the third-party payer, the providers are unlikely to receive payment for the services rendered and could potentially be charged with fraud.[4]

Examples of these types of regulations can be found in the Medicare system, which now requires that PTAs providing services to Medicare clients must (with some rare exceptions) have graduated from an accredited program and have passed a licensure examination, even if this is not a requirement of the state in which the PTA works.[15] Medicare also requires a higher level of supervision for PTAs in the private practice setting (direct supervision, meaning within the office suite[4]) than in other practice settings. In other settings, Medicare requires only general supervision, with supervisory visits required only every 30 days (however, state regulations regarding supervisory visits may differ). APTA members can find more information about Medicare's supervisory requirements on the "Medicare Payment and Reimbursement" page of the APTA website.[16]

Supervision of Students

The APTA and Medicare have regulations that apply to the supervision of PT and PTA students during their clinical experiences. The APTA has identified "direct supervision" as the level required for supervision of PT and PTA students. According to the position statement on levels of supervision, the APTA expects that the "physical therapist is physically present and immediately available" when supervising a PT or PTA student.[9] The APTA has clarified that this means the PT is within the building, although not necessarily in the same room.[17] Note that this position does not mention the PTA who may be serving as a clinical instructor (CI). Another position, "Supervision of Student Physical Therapist Assistants," describes how a PTA student may be supervised by either a PT or a PT/PTA team.[11] This indicates that a PTA should never serve as a CI in isolation, just as a PTA cannot work independently in a clinic without PT supervision. However, PTAs are encouraged to serve as CIs, as evidenced by their inclusion in the APTA's Clinical Instructor Education and Credentialing Program (see Chapter 14).[18]

Medicare also addresses the topic of student supervision, although Medicare's requirements are less clearly defined than those of the APTA. Supervision requirements differ based on the setting and which Medicare component, Part A or Part B, is covering the service. Because the regulations are inconsistent and confusing to many clinicians, the APTA has a chart that reviews Medicare's varying requirements for student supervision. This chart is found in some APTA publications, such as the CI Education and Credentialing Course Manual, and is posted on the Medicare page of the APTA's website.[16]

Like the APTA, Medicare also states that a PT must provide supervision of students, and the use of PTAs as CIs as part of a PT/PTA supervisory team is encouraged.[19] State statutes may also address the issue of student supervision or may be silent on the topic. Because Medicare's regulations regarding student supervision in the clinical setting have changed multiple times in recent years, the reader is encouraged to use APTA's resources for the most up-to-date information on student supervision requirements.

Licensure Requirements for PTAs

As with the other regulations that pertain to the PTA, the specific requirements for obtaining and maintaining licensure or other type of state-required credential vary considerably from state to state. In the past few years, all of the states that previously did not oversee PTA services have updated their practice acts to include some type of regulation, but the variation in regulation between states continues. States that require a licensure examination use one that has been developed and regulated by the FSBPT. The **National Physical Therapy Examination (NPTE)** is used to ensure a minimum level of competence among those who pass it. It is computer-based and is proctored by a national testing service. The PTA examination consists of 200 questions representative of the skills and knowledge level required of entry-level PTAs. The requirements for being eligible to sit for the examination may vary from state to state. However, all of the states that require the NPTE use the same score required for passing the examination.[20] More information on the process of preparing for and taking the NPTE is presented in Chapter 14.

Other types of requirements that states *may* mandate for registration or licensure include the following:[5]

- Graduating from a CAPTE-accredited PTA program or other board-approved educational program. In some states, graduates of PT programs may also be eligible for PTA licensure.
- Taking a **jurisprudence examination.** This is a written and/or oral examination that asks questions specific to that state's practice act.
- Completing and clearing a criminal background check.
- Paying an initial application and licensure fee set by that state and an annual renewal fee thereafter.
- Demonstrating experience or education equivalent to that which would have been received in an accredited PTA program, if not a graduate of such a program (i.e., a clinician trained outside of the United States).
- Completing a required number of employment hours and/or continuing education units for renewal of licensure.

SUMMARY

It is critical that PTs and PTAs understand all of the different, sometimes contradictory, regulations that apply to direction and supervision of the PTA, including PTA students. State practice acts, APTA positions and standards, and insurance regulations all must be taken into consideration. Whereas state policy is legally binding and must always be followed, the APTA and third-party payer policies can affect interpretation of "best practice" and payment for services. Although all 50 states now have some type of PTA regulations in place, the requirements for initial and ongoing licensure are inconsistent. Because regulations vary among states, the APTA, and third-party payers, it is essential that PTs and PTAs stay informed about any changes in the regulations affecting their particular state and practice setting. The APTA and the Federation of State Boards of Physical Therapy provide numerous online resources to help clinicians with this task.

REFERENCES

1. American Physical Therapy Association. *Guide to Physical Therapist Practice 3.0*. Alexandria, VA: American Physical Therapy Association. http://guidetoptpractice.apta.org/. Updated 2014. Accessed July 6, 2015.
2. American Physical Therapy Association. Direction and supervision of the physical therapist assistant (HOD P06-05-18-26). http://www.apta.org/uploadedFiles/APTAorg/About_Us/Policies/Practice/DirectionSupervisionPTA.pdf. Updated 2012. Accessed August 13, 2015.
3. Scott RW. *Foundations of Physical Therapy.* New York, NY: McGraw-Hill; 2002:484.
4. Nicholson S. *The Physical Therapist's Business Practice and Legal Guide.* Sudbury, MA: Jones & Bartlett; 2008:399.
5. Federation of State Boards of Physical Therapy. Licensure reference guide. https://www.fsbpt.org/FreeResources/RegulatoryResources/LicensureReferenceGuide. Updated 2011. Accessed August 13, 2015.
6. Federation of State Boards of Physical Therapy. About us. https://www.fsbpt.org/AboutUs.aspx. Updated 2015. Accessed August 13, 2015.
7. Federation of State Boards of Physical Therapy. *The Model Practice Act for Physical Therapy: A Tool for Public Protection and Legislative Change.* 5th ed. Fairfax, VA: Federation of State Boards of Physical Therapy; 2011. https://www.fsbpt.org/Portals/0/documents/free-resources/MPA_5thEdition2011.pdf. Updated 2011. Accessed August 13, 2015.
8. American Physical Therapy Association. Standing rules of the American Physical Therapy Association. http://www.apta.org/uploadedFiles/APTAorg/About_Us/Policies/General/StandingRules.pdf. Updated 2011. Accessed August 14, 2015.
9. American Physical Therapy Association. Levels of supervision (HOD P06-00-15-26). http://www.apta.org/uploadedFiles/APTAorg/About_Us/Policies/Terminology/LevelsSupervision.pdf. Updated 2012. Accessed August 13, 2015.
10. American Physical Therapy Association. Student physical therapist provision of services. http://www.apta.org/uploadedFiles/APTAorg/About_Us/Policies/Practice/StudentPTProvisionServices.pdf. Updated 2012. Accessed August 13, 2015.

11. American Physical Therapy Association. Supervision of student physical therapist assistants. http://www.apta.org/uploadedFiles/APTAorg/About_Us/Policies/Practice/SupervisionStudentPTA.pdf. Updated 2012. Accessed August 13, 2015.

12. American Physical Therapy Association. Provision of physical therapy services and related tasks (HOD P06-00-17-28). http://www.apta.org/uploadedFiles/APTAorg/About_Us/Policies/Practice/ProvisionInterventions.pdf. Updated 2012. Accessed August 10, 2015.

13. Crosier J. PTAs today: PTA direction and supervision algorithms. *PT in Motion*. 2010;9.

14. American Physical Therapy Association. PTA patient care and supervision. http://www.apta.org/PTA/PatientCare/. Updated 2015. Accessed August 13, 2015.

15. Centers for Medicare & Medicaid Services. CMS manual system transmittal 88: therapy personnel qualifications and policies effective January 1, 2008. http://www.cms.hhs.gov/transmittals/downloads/R88BP.pdf. Updated 2008. Accessed August 14, 2015.

16. American Physical Therapy Association. Medicare payment and reimbursement. http://www.apta.org/Medicare/. Updated 2015. Accessed April 21, 2015.

17. Bezner J. Supervision and best practice. *PT Magazine*. 2001;9(12):22.

18. American Physical Therapy Association. Credentialed clinical instructor program. http://www.apta.org/CCIP/. Updated 2015. Accessed August 14, 2015.

19. Centers for Medicare & Medicaid Services. Medicare intermediary manual: transmittal 1872. http://www.cms.hhs.gov/transmittals/downloads/r1872a3.pdf. Updated 2003. Accessed August 14, 2015.

20. Federation of State Boards of Physical Therapy. *NPTE Candidate Handbook*. Fairfax, VA: Federation of State Boards of Physical Therapy; 2015. http://www.fsbpt.org/FreeResources/NPTECandidateHandbook.aspx. Updated 2015. Accessed August 14, 2015.

Name _____

REVIEW

1. If your state practice act had different requirements for PTA direction and supervision from what is stated in APTA documents, which would you have to follow? Why?

_____

_____

2. Define the following terms:

   a. Supervisory visit: _____

   _____

   b. Supervision ratio: _____

   _____

   c. APTA position: _____

   _____

3. Match the type of APTA-recommended supervision with the type of personnel to which it applies.

   _____ Direct personal supervision

   _____ Direct supervision

   _____ General supervision

   a. The PT is physically present and immediately available for direction and supervision. The PT will have direct contact with the patient/client during each visit.

   b. The PT is not required to be on site for direction and supervision but must be available at least by telecommunications.

   c. The PT or, where allowable by law, the PTA is physically present and immediately available to direct and supervise tasks that are related to patient/client management. The direction and supervision are continual throughout the time these tasks are performed.

(questions continue on page 74)

Application

Complete the following table to compare and contrast the different regulations that affect PTAs using your own state's guidelines for the state practice act regulations. Be as specific as you can concerning your state's requirements (avoid yes/no answers; indicate if the item is not addressed). Your instructor may add items to the first column, relevant to your state.

	State Practice Act	APTA Positions
Level of supervision required for PTA?		
Supervision ratio? (PT/PTA)		
Written proof of supervision required?		
Regular observation of PTA performing intervention (supervisory visit) required?		
Able to supervise PT aides/technicians?		
Tasks that PTAs are prohibited from performing?		
Requirement for supervision of students?		
Other requirements?		

Ethics and Ethical Behavior in Physical Therapy

5

CHAPTER OBJECTIVES

After reading this chapter, the reader will be able to:

- Define terms related to ethics and ethical theory.
- Identify categories of ethical issues in physical therapy.
- Describe key components of ethical behavior.
- Use the Code of Ethics and Standards of Ethical Conduct for the Physical Therapist Assistant of the American Physical Therapy Association (APTA) to give examples of specific ethical behaviors to be demonstrated by physical therapists (PTs) and physical therapist assistants (PTAs).
- Identify strategies for how students might continue development of their ethical behaviors.
- Describe a decision-making model that can be used to determine appropriate action when encountering ethical dilemmas.
- Identify APTA resources for ethical development.
- Describe the processes of the APTA in dealing with ethical complaints

KEY TERMS AND CONCEPTS

- Ethical dilemma
- Nonmaleficence
- Beneficence
- Justice
- Autonomy
- Fidelity
- Veracity
- Duty
- Academic integrity
- Moral sensitivity
- Moral judgment
- Moral motivation
- Moral character
- Moral courage
- Code of ethics
- Standards of Ethical Behavior for the Physical Therapist Assistant
- RIPS Model of Ethical Decision-Making
- APTA Ethics and Judicial Committee (EJC)

T ony, a PTA, works in the subacute unit of a skilled nursing facility where most patients are typically seen twice daily for physical therapy sessions of 30 minutes each. Most of the patients in the subacute unit have their room, board, and therapy services covered under Medicare Part A. One of these patients, Mr. Alvarez, is recovering from a total knee replacement, and he missed his therapy sessions yesterday because of nausea and vomiting. The nurses believe it was a reaction to pain medication and have cleared Mr. Alvarez for therapy today. As Tony leaves the physical therapy department to see Mr. Alvarez, the rehabilitation manager, Terry, tells him, "Try to get as many extra minutes in as you can today with Mr. Alvarez. We're behind in our estimated minutes for him and need to get in more to reach our predicted reimbursement level. We can do it, but you will probably need to see him for at least 45 minutes instead of 30 minutes each time today." Tony has Mr. Alvarez practice ambulating outside in the morning, which takes up the extra 15 minutes. During the afternoon session, it is raining, and after the usual 30-minute session, Tony is not sure what else to add to fill in the extra 15 minutes. Mr. Alvarez now has company and does not want to participate in any more therapy this afternoon. Tony is unsure how to proceed.

QUESTIONS TO CONSIDER

What is an ethical dilemma? Have Tony's actions up to this point been ethical? What about Terry's actions? What are Tony's choices for action now? Is one course of action more appropriate than others? Are there APTA documents or decision-making tools that could help Tony feel more confident in his choice of action?

T he previous chapter discusses legal regulations found in state practice acts that relate to direction and supervision of the PTA. Chapter 10 reviews additional legal principles and regulations that, although not specific to physical therapy, dictate the way in which physical therapy is practiced. Laws, however, are only one driving force for the behaviors and decision-making that occur in the clinical setting. Some legal statutes have "gray" areas in which one specific course of action in a given situation may not be overtly mandated, allowing multiple interpretations of how the law should be followed. In these and other situations, a chosen course of action might not be considered illegal, yet may feel "wrong," and one might struggle with how to justify one's actions if challenged. There are also situations in which, rather than having to make choices of "right versus wrong," a clinician may feel as if she were choosing between "right versus right." In these situations, there may not be a clear "best" course of action, but a choice must be made. The basis for how one handles these types of situations often has as much to do with the moral and ethical principles that one upholds as it does with following the letter of the law.

This chapter discusses common ethical principles that relate to the delivery of physical therapy services, examines how the practice of ethical decision-making has evolved throughout the history of the profession, reviews the documents that have been created by the APTA to direct the moral actions of its members, and highlights models that facilitate appropriate ethical decision-making in those situations in which the "right" choice is unclear or uncomfortable, or has the potential to place the decision maker in some type of personal or professional jeopardy.

Introduction to Ethics and Ethical Theory

FOR REFLECTION
FOR REFLECTION

- Think of a time when you had to make a difficult decision. What were some of the factors that made the decision difficult to make? How did the process of making this decision affect your emotions? Did it affect you physically? Who or what helped you to make the decision?

For many people, decision-making can be very stressful, especially if the decision is not clear-cut. Although ethics have been defined as the "philosophical reflection on questions of right or wrong,"[1] ethical decisions are rarely straightforward, and there is more to being ethical than just being able to do the right thing.[2] Ruth Purtilo, one of the first PTs to study ethical behavior within the profession, defines an **ethical dilemma** as a type of ethical situation in which a person has to choose between two potential courses of action. Both may be appropriate, but only one can be taken.[3] An issue that is a dilemma for one person may be an easy decision for another person, depending on beliefs and cultural background. In fact, what is considered unethical by one culture may be considered socially appropriate behavior by another.[4] For example, using someone's original work in a paper without crediting the author, considered to be plagiarism in the United States' dominant culture, may not be considered inappropriate in another culture that places more emphasis on group versus original work. It may be considered a sign of respect for the original author's work and might not be deemed improper.[5]

As the role of the PT has evolved into that of an autonomous practitioner, the complexity of potential ethical situations has increased.[6,7] Before looking at the types of issues faced in physical therapy today, it may be helpful to review a few concepts and terms related to the study of ethics. Following the model used by Swisher, this book assumes that the terms "ethical" and "moral" can be used interchangeably.[6]

Ethics Theory and Terminology

Four basic ethical concepts have direct application to the delivery of quality health-care services.[8] Most people entering a medical profession have heard of the Hippocratic oath that, in part, states *prium non nocere,* or "first, do no harm." The concept of doing no harm is described by the term **nonmaleficence.** Along those same lines, what caregivers strive to do in their daily work falls into the category of **beneficence,** "doing good" for others. The other basic principles include **justice,** a matter of dealing with all people in the same fair manner, and **autonomy,** the right of people to have choices and to make their own decisions regarding those choices.[1,8] Other related ethical concepts include **fidelity** (keeping commitments made to others), **veracity** (the obligation to be truthful in words and actions), and **duty** (responsibilities owed to others).[8]

All these terms describe positive ideals. The challenges come when one or more of these ideals are in conflict with others. For example, the benefits of using a physical therapy technique such as active assistive range of motion after joint replacement surgery (doing "good") may conflict with increased pain perceived by the patient (doing "harm"). The patient may refuse her therapy (the right of autonomy), and if the patient is perceived as being rude or difficult in doing so, the clinician may not use the same amount of effort in attempting to convince her to participate as she might with a patient who refuses in a more polite manner (potentially an issue of justice). In this type of situation, one must decide whether the merits of one course of action outweigh the merits of another.

In making these decisions, people usually seek some type of justification for choosing one option instead of another. The concept of providing a rationale for one's actions should be a familiar one to the reader who is currently in a physical therapy academic program. Students are frequently asked to provide rationales for their actions during practical examinations as a way for their instructors to connect students' thinking to their actions. This is not unique to physical therapy education. People often are asked to give a rationale for why they act (or do not act) in a given manner, and generations of philosophers have debated the merits of various ethical theories that have been applied to human behavior, in attempts to justify why people follow one course of action rather than another. In reviewing the most familiar, time-honored philosophies, Gabard and Martin indicate that no one theory is better than another, and all can be valuable in organizing one's beliefs and subsequent actions as long as they are compatible with an individual's own moral convictions.[9] The accompanying table shows a synopsis of some of the most common theoretical models.

Types of Ethical Problems

Most clinicians would probably say that they always try to act in the best interests of their patients, but today's clinical environment has become more challenging, and it is not unusual for a student to go out on her first clinical experience and witness one or more examples of situations in which ethical principles may have been compromised.[2] Being aware of the ethical issues its practitioners face is expected of a maturing profession,[6,10,11] but physical therapy has only recently begun to take a more in-depth look at this issue. Triezenberg identified three categories of ethical issues facing physical therapy providers:[11]

Theory[1,9]	Focus	Description
Rights ethics	Human rights	Conduct is right when it supports the fundamental morally valid entitlements of others, often divided into liberty rights and welfare rights.
Duty ethics (deontological)	Duties	Individuals should always act in a prescribed manner based on rights of and duties to others.
Utilitarian	Consequences	Actions should produce the most good for the most people.
Act utilitarian	Actions	Identify all the possible actions in a situation, and choose the one that maximizes good overall.
Rule utilitarian	Rules	Actions are right when they conform to rules that maximize good.
Virtue ethics	Character traits	Individuals should strive to demonstrate desirable patterns of behaviors (virtues) instead of undesirable ones (vices).
Religious ethics	Worldview	Moral judgments are justified based on guidance and commandments of a higher power.
Pragmatism	Context	Look at individual situations and paradigms; find the best way to honor all involved values.

FOR REFLECTION

- Do any of the ethical theories listed in the table best reflect the way you handle decision-making situations? Can you think of a time when this theory did not work for you?

- **Patient rights/patient welfare concerns:** Issues related to confidentiality, informed consent, sexual misconduct of providers, discrimination against patients, and using human subjects in research

- **Professional issues:** Concerns regarding appropriate competence, utilization of services, supervision of support personnel, safety of the work environment, and reporting misconduct
- **Business/economic issues:** Issues related to cost justification and fraud prevention, concerns with appropriate advertising, product endorsements, and business relationships

Often, the concerns are not related to what Triezenberg and Davis refer to as "headlining issues such as cloning or end-of-life decision-making"; rather, they are more often related to daily patient/provider interaction.[2]

FOR REFLECTION
FOR REFLECTION

- Identify an example of unethical behavior that might occur in each of the preceding categories related to the role of the PTA.

Developing Ethical Behaviors

Scott maintains that each PT and PTA must develop her own framework for determining the weight of ethical issues and internal mechanisms for assessing her professional behavior.[12] The most effective way for the profession of physical therapy to maximize this individual development is to begin the process while clinicians are still students.[2] For most physical therapy students, their first exposure to ethics in their academic curriculum may be related to the concept of **academic integrity.** All academic institutions have policies concerning expectations for student behavior related to doing one's own work. Additionally, students may be asked to sign a document in which they agree to certain standards of behavior in the classroom or clinical setting. In 2004, the APTA House of Delegates passed a guideline to promote the use of a professional oath for PT students.[13] Although this was not designed for the PTA student, many schools have begun to use some type of conduct code in an attempt to promote ethical behavior in students.

The term "ethical behavior" has been used somewhat generically up to this point in the chapter. But what exactly is meant by ethical behavior? Triezenberg and Davis built on the work of Rest[14] by proposing that ethical behavior includes the following four characteristics:[2]

- **Moral sensitivity:** Being able to identify a situation with ethical overtones
- **Moral judgment:** Being able to analyze a situation and make an appropriate decision
- **Moral motivation:** Distinguishing which moral factors are more relative than others
- **Moral character:** Having the courage to act on the decisions one makes

Purtilo discusses the characteristic of **moral courage** as being ready to take action in stressful situations "in order to uphold something of great moral value."[15] Davis also refers to moral courage as being "deeper than the action itself … flow(ing) from a generous and caring heart."[16]

Can students actually learn these behaviors? Educators disagree over where and how ethics should be taught in the academic curriculum.[17] In recent years, many educators have identified strategies they believe have enabled students to develop a better sense of their own ethical philosophy and have made them better equipped to identify ethical issues in the clinical setting. Although the profession is not moving away from teaching ethical theory, ethical principles seem to have more meaning for students when applied to cases they discuss in the classroom or experience in the clinical setting.[18,19] Many experts encourage the use of journals or other types of writing assignments to develop students' self-reflection skills in ethics.[18,20] Reviewing and discussing the Code of Ethics for Physical Therapists and Standards of Ethical Conduct for the Physical Therapist Assistant (see next section of this chapter), the "Professionalism in Physical Therapy: Core Values" document (Chapter 1), and the Professional Behaviors assessment tool (Chapter 12) can also help students to integrate these principles into their personal value systems.[18] Developing class codes of conduct and participating in in-service learning activities, combined with discussion and journaling, are other ways to provide actual context to the theoretical concepts of ethics.[2]

FOR REFLECTION

- Do you believe that ethical behavior can be taught? Why or why not? Up to this point in your life, what influences have had the greatest effect on the development of your ethical behavior?

Evolution of Ethical Behaviors in Physical Therapy

As mentioned in Chapter 1, one of the hallmarks of a profession is that it has some type of document that describes the behaviors to which members of the profession are expected to adhere, generally referred to as a **code of ethics.** The need for ethical codes comes from the duty-based ethical theory of the German philosopher Immanuel Kant, outlining the duties of those in a profession.[21] The physical therapy profession's first Code of Ethics and Discipline was adopted by the APTA in 1935.[22] The PTA version, **Standards of Ethical Conduct for the Physical Therapist Assistant,** was added in 1981.[23] However, as physical therapist practice has changed over the years, so have the expectations and definitions of ethical behavior, and these core documents have evolved along with those expectations.

Professional codes represent a social contract between the profession and the public it serves.[9] However, the early versions of physical therapy codes of ethics had less to do with the patient and more to do with how PTs should behave in their interactions with physicians (which was to act in a deferential manner toward them).[22] As physical therapist practice has evolved, the ethical philosophies have changed. Purtilo describes how the profession has evolved through three different periods of ethical identity. She calls the early days a period of "self-identity," in which physical therapy was merely trying to establish itself among other fields in health care. In the 1950s, as patient autonomy and patient rights became more prominent, the profession moved into a period of "patient identity," and the patient became the focus of ethical consideration. Most recently, PTs and PTAs have begun to recognize their obligations to society as a whole (Purtilo's period of "societal identity"), and the profession has begun to debate ethical issues beyond those relating specifically to direct patient care.[22]

Two documents, the Code of Ethics for the Physical Therapist and the Standards of Ethical Conduct for the Physical Therapist Assistant, have evolved to reflect these changes. They were most recently modified by the APTA House of Delegates in 2009, with significant updates in language and expectations to reflect current practice. Both documents have accompanying guides that provide context and serve to interpret the standards. Many of the original examples of behaviors included in previous versions of these guides have now been merged into their respective code and standards documents, creating a more comprehensive document for each role.[24]

Why are there separate versions of these documents? The difference in titles is most likely related to the belief, as described in Chapter 1, that the role of the PTA does not meet the historical criteria for a "professional," and as such, a "code of ethics" would be inappropriate. Differences in the documents themselves relate to the higher level of accountability required of the PT and to the PT's extensive scope of practice and multiple roles.[25] Additionally, following each principle found in the Code of Ethics for the Physical Therapist is a listing of the core values that relate to that specific principle (because the core values document was written to reflect the PT's role rather than the PTA's, these connections are not included in the Standards of Ethical Conduct).

The two documents are much more alike, however, than they are different. Each document mandates behavioral actions (as indicated by use of the word "shall" in each, which implies a duty or obligation to fulfill[26]) in eight categories. In the PT's Code of Ethics, the categories are called "principles," whereas in the PTA version they are called "standards." Much of the language in the Standards of Ethical Conduct for the Physical Therapist Assistant is identical to that in the PT's Code of Ethics. Areas in which they differ reflect the different responsibilities of the two roles, not any difference in the overall level of ethical behavior. Both documents now have more specific descriptions and examples that reflect the current challenges and responsibilities of today's clinical environment, making it easier for clinicians in both roles to determine whether they are upholding the expectations set for them. Both also place a greater emphasis on establishing effective relationships with others, following ethical business practices, and advocating for the needs of society as a whole.[27]

FOR REFLECTION

- In arguing that PTAs should be held no less accountable than PTs in the area of ethics, some people maintain that the APTA should have only one document dictating ethical behavior. Do you agree or disagree with this? Why?

Standards of Ethical Conduct for the Physical Therapist Assistant (HOD S06-09-20-18)

Preamble

The Standards of Ethical Conduct for the Physical Therapist Assistant (Standards of Ethical Conduct) delineate the ethical obligations of all physical therapist assistants as determined by the House of Delegates of the American Physical Therapy Association (APTA). The Standards of Ethical Conduct provide a foundation for conduct to which all physical therapist assistants shall adhere. Fundamental to the Standards of Ethical Conduct is the special obligation of physical therapist assistants to enable patients/clients to achieve greater independence, health and wellness, and enhanced quality of life. No document that delineates ethical standards can address every situation. Physical therapist assistants are encouraged to seek additional advice or consultation in instances where the guidance of the Standards of Ethical Conduct may not be definitive.

Standards

Standard #1: Physical therapist assistants shall respect the inherent dignity, and rights, of all individuals.

1A. Physical therapist assistants shall act in a respectful manner toward each person regardless of age, gender, race, nationality, religion, ethnicity, social or economic status, sexual orientation, health condition, or disability.

1B. Physical therapist assistants shall recognize their personal biases and shall not discriminate against others in the provision of physical therapy services.

Standard #2: Physical therapist assistants shall be trustworthy and compassionate in addressing the rights and needs of patients/clients.

2A. Physical therapist assistants shall act in the best interests of patients/clients over the interests of the physical therapist assistant.

2B. Physical therapist assistants shall provide physical therapy interventions with compassionate and caring behaviors that incorporate the individual and cultural differences of patients/clients.

2C. Physical therapist assistants shall provide patients/clients with information regarding the interventions they provide.

2D. Physical therapist assistants shall protect confidential patient/client information and, in collaboration with the physical therapist, may disclose confidential information to appropriate authorities only when allowed or as required by law.

Standard #3: Physical therapist assistants shall make sound decisions in collaboration with the physical therapist and within the boundaries established by laws and regulations.

3A. Physical therapist assistants shall make objective decisions in the patient's/client's best interest in all practice settings.

3B. Physical therapist assistants shall be guided by information about best practice regarding physical therapy interventions.

3C. Physical therapist assistants shall make decisions based upon their level of competence and consistent with patient/client values.

(box continues on page 84)

Standards of Ethical Conduct for the Physical Therapist Assistant (HOD S06-09-20-18) (continued)

3D. Physical therapist assistants shall not engage in conflicts of interest that interfere with making sound decisions.

3E. Physical therapist assistants shall provide physical therapy services under the direction and supervision of a physical therapist and shall communicate with the physical therapist when patient/client status requires modifications to the established plan of care.

Standard #4: Physical therapist assistants shall demonstrate integrity in their relationships with patients/clients, families, colleagues, students, other health care providers, employers, payers, and the public.

4A. Physical therapist assistants shall provide truthful, accurate, and relevant information and shall not make misleading representations.

4B. Physical therapist assistants shall not exploit persons over whom they have supervisory, evaluative or other authority (e.g., patients/clients, students, supervisees, research participants, or employees).

4C. Physical therapist assistants shall discourage misconduct by health care professionals and report illegal or unethical acts to the relevant authority, when appropriate.

4D. Physical therapist assistants shall report suspected cases of abuse involving children or vulnerable adults to the supervising physical therapist and the appropriate authority, subject to law.

4E. Physical therapist assistants shall not engage in any sexual relationship with any of their patients/clients, supervisees, or students.

4F. Physical therapist assistants shall not harass anyone verbally, physically, emotionally, or sexually.

Standard #5: Physical therapist assistants shall fulfill their legal and ethical obligations.

5A. Physical therapist assistants shall comply with applicable local, state, and federal laws and regulations.

5B. Physical therapist assistants shall support the supervisory role of the physical therapist to ensure quality care and promote patient/client safety.

5C. Physical therapist assistants involved in research shall abide by accepted standards governing protection of research participants.

5D. Physical therapist assistants shall encourage colleagues with physical, psychological, or substance-related impairments that may adversely impact their professional responsibilities to seek assistance or counsel.

5E. Physical therapist assistants who have knowledge that a colleague is unable to perform their professional responsibilities with reasonable skill and safety shall report this information to the appropriate authority.

Standard #6: Physical therapist assistants shall enhance their competence through the lifelong acquisition and refinement of knowledge, skills, and abilities.

6A. Physical therapist assistants shall achieve and maintain clinical competence.

6B. Physical therapist assistants shall engage in lifelong learning consistent with changes in their roles and responsibilities and advances in the practice of physical therapy.

Standards of Ethical Conduct for the Physical Therapist Assistant (HOD S06-09-20-18) (continued)

6C. Physical therapist assistants shall support practice environments that support career development and lifelong learning.

Standard #7: Physical therapist assistants shall support organizational behaviors and business practices that benefit patients/clients and society.

7A. Physical therapist assistants shall promote work environments that support ethical and accountable decision-making.

7B. Physical therapist assistants shall not accept gifts or other considerations that influence or give an appearance of influencing their decisions.

7C. Physical therapist assistants shall fully disclose any financial interest they have in products or services that they recommend to patients/clients.

7D. Physical therapist assistants shall ensure that documentation for their interventions accurately reflects the nature and extent of the services provided.

7E. Physical therapist assistants shall refrain from employment arrangements, or other arrangements, that prevent physical therapist assistants from fulfilling ethical obligations to patients/clients.

Standard #8: Physical therapist assistants shall participate in efforts to meet the health needs of people locally, nationally, or globally.

8A. Physical therapist assistants shall support organizations that meet the health needs of people who are economically disadvantaged, uninsured, and underinsured.

8B. Physical therapist assistants shall advocate for people with impairments, activity limitations, participation restrictions, and disabilities in order to promote their participation in community and society.

8C. Physical therapist assistants shall be responsible stewards of health care resources by collaborating with physical therapists in order to avoid overutilization or underutilization of physical therapy services.

8D. Physical therapist assistants shall educate members of the public about the benefits of physical therapy.

Using an Ethical Decision-Making Model

When faced with making a decision in a situation that involves ethical components, it is difficult to keep emotions from coming into play. However, this is not always inappropriate. Greenfield believes that "moral emotion," emotion linked to the welfare of society or another person that helps alert one to a moral issue, can be either a positive or negative influence on moral behavior. He believes that emotion, as a naturally occurring physiological process, should be used along with reason in ethical decision-making.[21] However, it is often easier to make a decision that is based less on emotion and more on facts. One model for doing so was recently developed by Swisher, Arslanian, and Davis. Based on the work of Glaser,[28] this model, the **RIPS Model of Ethical Decision-Making** (see the accompanying table) offers "a rational, linear approach to resolving an ethical problem."[29] The acronym RIPS represents the components to be analyzed in the first of four steps of the decision-making process: realm, individual process, and situation.

In which REALM is the problem occurring? (Listed from least complex to most complex)	Which type of INDIVIDUAL PROCESS is required of me? (The behavior that needs to be demonstrated)	What kind of ethical SITUATION is involved? (Should be connected to the type of process selected)
Individual: *focusing on the rights of the patient, duties of individuals, and relationships between people*	Moral sensitivity	Issue/problem: *a value is challenged.*
	Moral judgment	Dilemma: *two alternative courses of action may each be considered right.*
	Moral motivation	
Organizational/institutional: *dealing with policies and systems that support an institution*	Moral courage	Distress: *right course of action is clear but can't or not allowed to do it.*
	(Refer to definitions presented previously in chapter)	
Societal: *relating to the common good of all*		Temptation: *a benefit exists for doing wrong instead of right.*
		Silence: *values are challenged but no one is addressing it or taking action.*

From Swisher LL, Arslanian LE, Davis CM. The Realm-Individual Process-Situation (RIPS) Model of Ethical Decision-Making. *HPA Resource.* 2005;5(3):1, with permission.

FOR REFLECTION

- Go back to the scenario in the beginning of this chapter. Using the preceding table, identify the *realm, individual process,* and *situation* occurring in this scenario.

According to the developers of this model, following the steps of this framework encourages more deliberate analysis prior to decision-making and allows the decision maker to "walk all the way around" the multiple sides of an ethical issue. The developers recognize that it is a somewhat "rational, linear approach" that will not work for all ethical issues and does not always allow for emotion or for the relevant experiences of others.[29] However, for those who may struggle with the process of making difficult decisions, the model may provide a more systematic way to recognize and consider all factors. The application of this model to real-life examples is frequently featured in a monthly column, "Ethics in Practice" (discussed below), in the APTA magazine *PT in Motion*.

Step 1: Recognizing and defining the ethical issue: Gather the factual information, describe issue, identify its **Realm, Individual Process,** and **Situation.**

Step 2: Reflecting on it: What are possible responses? Do responses match with the issue's realm? Can you determine whether something is right or wrong? Ask yourself:

Is it illegal?
Does it "feel" wrong? (Pay attention to your "gut reaction.")
Would you want your action to be on the front page of the newspaper?
Would your parent do this?
Does the action violate the APTA's Code of Ethics, Standards of Ethical Conduct, or core values?

Step 3: Deciding what to do: Use rule-based *(follow rules)*, ends-based *(determine consequences of actions in terms of good/harm to others)*, and/or care-based *(think about relationships with others)* approach.

Step 4: Implementing, evaluating, and reassessing the decision: Was your initial analysis correct? What did you learn? How can you better prepare yourself for future issues?

From Swisher LL, Arslanian LE, Davis CM. The Realm-Individual-Process-Situation (RIPS) Model of Ethical Decision-Making. *HPA Resource.* 2005;5(3):1, with permission.

Resources for Supporting Ethical Behavior and Development

Why is it essential to be able to deal with ethical issues appropriately? Students tend to place greater emphasis and importance on the factual knowledge learned in the "hard sciences" as opposed to that which is more "behavioral" in nature.[2] However, Sisola found that students who demonstrated stronger moral reasoning skills also tended to demonstrate stronger levels of overall performance in the clinical environment. She believes that demonstrating the ability to recognize and deal with ethical issues is a key component of demonstrating clinical competence.[30] Scott agrees that clinicians must stay informed of developments in health law and health-care ethics as a component of maintaining one's clinical competence. One way that he encourages clinicians to do this is by participating in regular continuing education opportunities on these topics.[12]

The APTA has a number of resources available to keep members current on ethical practice. The **APTA Ethics and Judicial Committee (EJC)** is charged with educating members about ethical practice and the documents that regulate it,[31] and they accomplish this in many ways. The APTA website includes the page "Ethics and Professionalism," which contains links to the APTA's core ethics documents and other resources and documents compiled by the EJC to assist members and consumers to deal with suspected violations or ethical complaints filed against them. Another section of this page contains links to educational resources for members, including past EJC decisions, information about the disciplinary process, continuing education opportunities, links to the RIPS model, and copies of presentations and articles on legal and ethical issues.[32]

Another excellent resource for learning how to apply the profession's core ethical documents is the APTA's monthly publication, *PT in Motion*. The magazine features a regular column called "Ethics in Practice." The goal of the column, written by a former member of the EJC, is to "make explicit the central role of ethical analysis and behavior in the everyday practice of physical therapy."[24] The column uses real-life scenarios in which to consider application of the Code of Ethics and the Standards of Ethical Conduct, frequently using the RIPS model. The magazine is included as part of annual APTA membership and is available in hard copy or electronically.

FOR REFLECTION
FOR REFLECTION

- Have you witnessed any ethical dilemmas in the clinical setting? If you haven't yet had any clinical experiences, think about any observation opportunities in which you participated, or even something that occurred when you were a patient. Did the people involved handle the situation as you would have done? Discuss with a classmate what you might have done similarly or differently.

Ethical Violations

When an APTA member is suspected of an ethical violation, the complaint is first investigated at the state level by the chapter president and the chapter's ethics committee; if not dismissed there, it then moves to the national level, where it is addressed by the EJC.[33] The EJC is responsible for processing reported Code of Ethics/Standards of Ethical Behavior violations and makes final decisions on disciplinary action involving members.[31] The possible EJC decision outcomes regarding an ethics charge include dismissal of the charges, issuing a written reprimand (a nonpublic sanction), suspending the violator's APTA membership privileges, or expelling the violator from the association.[33]

SUMMARY

In this author's experience, it is not unusual for students to report that ethical dilemmas were infrequently noted during the course of their clinical experiences. However, it is not accurate to assume that the absence of problems means that an individual is not dealing with ethical issues. As health-care providers, everything done in interaction with patients/clients has an ethical or a moral component.[2] The ethical decision-making that is occurring during those interactions needs to be viewed as part of the overall clinical decision-making, not as a separate component of care.[34] By becoming more aware of the components of ethics and the examples of appropriate ethical behavior as described in the Standards and by using decision-making models that promote objective analysis of one's choices, PTAs can more easily incorporate this component of decision-making into their daily interactions with patients and others.

REFERENCES

1. Swisher LL, Krueger-Brophy C. *Legal and Ethical Issues in Physical Therapy.* Boston, MA: Butterworth-Heinemann; 1998:231.
2. Triezenberg HL, Davis C. Beyond the code of ethics: educating physical therapists for their role as moral agents. *J Phys Ther Educ.* 2000;14(3):48-58.
3. Purtilo RB. *Ethical Dimensions in the Health Professions.* 4th ed. Philadelphia, PA: Elsevier Saunders; 2005:346.
4. Lattanzi JB, Purnell LD. *Developing Cultural Competence in Physical Therapy Practice.* Philadelphia, PA: FA Davis; 2006:417.
5. Howard R. *Standing in the Shadow of Giants: Plagiarists, Authors, Collaborators.* Washington State University Library. Cultural Perspectives on Plagiarism. Web site. http://www.wsulibs.wsu.edu/library-instruction/plagiarism/cultural-perspectives. Published 1999. Updated 2015. Accessed August 14, 2015.
6. Swisher LL. A retrospective analysis of ethics knowledge in physical therapy (1970-2000). *Phys Ther.* 2002;82(7):692-706. http://search.ebscohost.com/login.aspx?direct=true&db=rzh&AN=2002134844&site=ehost-live.
7. Guccione A. Ethical issues in physical therapy practice: a survey of physical therapists in New England. *Phys Ther.* 1980;60:1264-1272.
8. Kornblau BL, Burkhardt A. *Ethics in Rehabilitation: A Clinical Perspective.* 2nd ed. Thorofare, NJ: SLACK; 2012.
9. Gabard DL, Martin MW. *Physical Therapy Ethics.* 2nd ed. Philadelphia, PA: FA Davis; 2011:188.
10. Stiller C. Exploring the ethos of the physical therapy profession in the United States: social, cultural, and historical influences and their relationship to education. *J Phys Ther Educ.* 2000;14(3).
11. Triezenberg H. The identification of ethical issues in physical therapy practice. *Phys Ther.* 1996;76(10):1097-1108.
12. Scott RW. Supporting professional development: understanding the interplay between helath law and professional ethics. *J Phys Ther Educ.* 2000;14(3):17-19.
13. Wise D. Professionalism in physical therapy: an oath for physical therapists. *J Phys Ther Educ.* 2014;28(1):58-63.
14. Rest JR. *Moral Development: Advances in Theory and Research.* New York, NY: Praeger; 1986.
15. Purtilo RB. Moral courage in times of change: visions for the future. *J Phys Ther Educ.* 2000;14(3):4-6.
16. Davis C. Educating adult health professionals for moral action: in search of moral courage. In: Purtilo RB, Jensen GM, Brasic Royeen C, eds. *Educating for*

Moral Action: A Sourcebook in Health and Rehabilitation Ethics. Vol 20. Philadelphia, PA: FA Davis; 2005:215-224.

17. Sisola S. Integrating theories and practices of adult teaching and learning: implications for ethics education. In: Purtilo RB, Jensen GM, Brasic Royeen C, eds. *Educating for Moral Action: A Sourcebook in Health and Rehabilitation Ethics.* Philadelphia, PA: FA Davis; 2005:239-249.

18. Jensen GM, Richert AE. Reflection on the teaching of ethics in physical therapist education: integrating cases, theory, and learning. *J Phys Ther Educ.* 2005;19(3): 78-85. http://search.ebscohost.com/login.aspx?direct=true&db=rzh&AN =2009123404&site=ehost-live.

19. Venglar M, Theall M. Case-based ethics education in physical therapy. *J Scholarship Teaching Learning.* 2007;7(1):64-76.

20. Romanello M. The "ethic of care" in physical therapy practice and education: challenges and opportunities. *J Phys Ther Educ.* 2000;14(3):20-25.

21. Greenfield B. The role of emotions in ethical decision making: implications for physical therapist education. *J Phys Ther Educ.* 2007;21(1):14-21. http:// search.ebscohost.com/login.aspx?direct=true&db=rzh&AN=2009598655&site =ehost-live.

22. Purtilo R. A time to harvest, a time to sow: ethics for a shifting landscape. *Phys Ther.* 2000;80(11):1112-1119. http://search.ebscohost.com/login.aspx?direct=true &db=keh&AN=3913514&site=ehost-live.

23. American Physical Therapy Association. Standards of ethical conduct for the physical therapist assistant. http://www.apta.org/uploadedFiles/APTAorg/About _Us/Policies/Ethics/StandardsEthicalConductPTA.pdf. Updated 2015. Accessed August 13, 2015.

24. Kirsch NR. Bringing us up to code. *PT Motion.* 2009;1(1):64-66. http:// search.ebscohost.com/login.aspx?direct=true&db=rzh&AN=2010439178&site =ehost-live.

25. American Physical Therapy Association. *Guide to Physical Therapist Practice 3.0.* Alexandria, VA: American Physical Therapy Association. http://guidetoptpractice.apta.org/. Updated 2014. Accessed July 6, 2015.

26. American Physical Therapy Association. Implications for motion language. http://www.apta.org/HOD/MotionProcess/. Updated 2015. Accessed August 14, 2015.

27. Kirsch NR. New and improved. *PT Motion.* 2009;1(2):50-55. http:// search.ebscohost.com/login.aspx?direct=true&db=rzh&AN=2010466333&site =ehost-live.

28. Glaser J. Three realms of ethics: an integrating map of ethics for the future. In: Purtilo RB, Jensen GM, Brasic Royeen C, eds. *Educating for Moral Action: A Sourcebook in Health and Rehabilitation Ethics.* Philadelphia, PA: FA Davis; 2005:169-184.

29. Swisher LL, Arslanian LE, Davis CM. The Realm-Individual-Process-Situation (RIPS) Model of Ethical Decision-Making. *HPA Resource.* 2005;5(3):1. http:// search.ebscohost.com/login.aspx?direct=true&db=rzh&AN=2009089605&site =ehost-live.

30. Sisola SW. Moral reasoning as a predictor of clinical practice: the development of physical therapy students across the professional curriculum. *J Phys Ther Educ*. 2000;14(3):26-34.

31. American Physical Therapy Association. APTA bylaws article X: committees and councils. http://www.apta.org/uploadedFiles/APTAorg/About_Us/Policies/General/Bylaws.pdf. Updated 2014. Accessed August 14, 2015.

32. American Physical Therapy Association. Ethics & professionalism. http://www.apta.org/EthicsProfessionalism/. Updated 2015. Accessed August 14, 2015.

33. American Physical Therapy Association. Resolving disputes or complaints. http://www.apta.org/Ethics/Disputes/. Updated 2014. Accessed August 15, 2015.

34. Dalton A, Arslanian L, Davis C, et al. Applying ethics to real world situations: a roundtable discussion offers suggestions on ways PTs can address ethical dilemmas in their daily activities. *PT Magazine*. 2005;13(3):40. http://search.ebscohost.com/login.aspx?direct=true&db=rzh&AN=2005076012&site=ehost-live.

Name _____

REVIEW

1. An ethical issue often involves choices of "right versus right." What is meant by this?

   _____

   _____

   _____

   _____

2. List and describe the three categories of ethical issues that affect the delivery of PT services.

   _____

   _____

   _____

3. Define five characteristics that are major components of ethical behavior.

   _____

   _____

   _____

   _____

   _____

4. List three methods that might be used with students to help them develop their ethical behaviors.

   _____

   _____

   _____

   _____

(questions continue on page 94)

Application

1. Review the Standards of Ethical Conduct for the Physical Therapist Assistant and identify the standard(s) that should drive the PTA's behavior in each of the following situations:

   ▪ A patient gives her a $100 bill "for a job well done."

   _____

   ▪ The PTA works part-time at an outpatient clinic and part-time at a fitness center as a personal trainer where she gets paid a bonus for every referral she obtains. The PTA often suggests that patients continue to see her at the fitness center after being discharged from the outpatient clinic.

   _____

   ▪ The PTA suspects that a colleague is working under the influence of drugs.

   _____

   ▪ The PTA refuses to work with a patient who has AIDS.

   _____

2. Imagine you are working as a PTA. You stop to say goodbye to a patient who has met her goals and is scheduled to be discharged tomorrow. The patient tells you that her daughter is ill and will not be available to stay with her after discharge, as previously planned, until later in the week. The patient tells you she is afraid to stay alone and asks you whether she can remain at the facility until her daughter is feeling better. You explain that she can stay, but her room and board will no longer be covered by insurance because she has been discharged from physical therapy. The patient then asks you whether she can resume physical therapy "for just a couple more days" to get her room and board covered.

   Using the Standards of Ethical Conduct for the Physical Therapist Assistant and the RIPS Model of Ethical Decision-Making as guides, follow the succeeding steps, and answer the questions in each step to determine how you might deal with this ethical situation.

Step 1: Recognizing and defining the ethical issue:
Identify the:

- Realm
- Individual Process
- Situation

Step 2: Reflecting on it:
What are possible responses?
Do your responses match with the issue's realm?

Step 3: Deciding what to do:
Determine a course of action.
Does your course of action follow a rule-based, ends-based, or care-based approach?

Step 4: Implementing, evaluating, and reassessing the decision:
What would be a positive outcome for this scenario? A negative outcome?
What can you learn from this situation?
Were there alternative ways of appropriately dealing with this situation?

6

The Patient–Physical Therapist Assistant Relationship

CHAPTER OBJECTIVES

After reading this chapter, the reader will be able to:

- Give examples of patient rights that are supported by law and the American Physical Therapy Association (APTA) policies.
- Provide rationales to explain why patients may have difficulty asserting their rights.
- Discuss the responsibility of the physical therapist assistant (PTA) in ensuring that patient rights are being maintained.
- Describe the intent of the Health Insurance Portability and Accountability Act.
- Explain how behavioral and psychosocial factors influence the patient-PTA relationship.
- Describe how the PTA's personal and professional values can affect his role as a health-care provider.
- Discuss the role of communication in developing rapport with patients.
- Give examples of verbal and nonverbal communication (speaking and listening) skills required for developing rapport with patients.
- Discuss how culture influences one's preferred communication style.
- Discuss appropriate ways to minimize the communication barriers related to language.
- Identify strategies to facilitate improved communication in times of conflict.

KEY TERMS AND CONCEPTS

- Patient Bill of Rights
- Informed consent
- The Health Insurance Portability and Accountability Act (HIPAA)
- Stages of grief
- Empathy
- Empowerment
- Advocacy
- Accountability
- Rapport
- Open-ended questions
- Active listening
- "I" messages

Matthew, a PTA working in an outpatient setting, is reviewing his schedule for the day. His supervising physical therapist (PT), Mya, tells him, "Your first patient this afternoon, Mr. Erickson, can be kind of difficult. Last time when he was here, he said he might not come back because the exercises we give him are too hard for him to do. I think he just isn't very motivated. But his daughter brings him here, and she says she's going to keep bringing him to physical therapy, whether he wants to come or not. I thought maybe you would have better luck connecting with him than I did." Matthew is apprehensive about working with Mr. Erickson and wonders whether he'll be able to get Mr. Erickson to participate. He asks Mya, "What should I do if he won't cooperate with the exercises? We can't force him to do physical therapy!"

QUESTIONS TO CONSIDER

What rights do patients have in the patient/provider relationship? Who is responsible for ensuring that the patient's rights are maintained? What psychosocial factors can interfere with the patient's ability to fully participate in physical therapy? What communication strategies can be used to ensure that the patient understands his rights and responsibilities regarding physical therapy and to encourage his full participation in a given intervention session?

Physical therapy, in most cases, is quite demanding for patients. It is often the clinician's role to help the patient improve his ability to perform tasks that currently are painful to do or can be done only with assistance. Many of the exercises and activities used by the PT or PTA to help improve a patient's functional abilities and overall health conditions (for example, those used to help improve range of motion, balance, coordination, strength, or endurance) may cause a patient to become anxious or apprehensive because of their challenging nature and potential for causing discomfort or fatigue. Many clinicians have initiated an intervention session only to have the patient grimace, groan, or otherwise indicate reluctance to participate. It takes talent on the part of the PT or PTA to gain the patient's full trust and cooperation in a manner that respects the patient's rights and acknowledges the difficulties of the patient's unique situation, yet pushes the patient enough to make gains toward his goals and outcomes. This chapter addresses the knowledge and skills that are necessary for facilitating the development of this type of relationship.

The Rights of the Patient

In the early days of medicine, health care was generally provided in a model of "paternalism" in which the care providers held complete decision-making power over what was done to the patient.[1] This model prevailed until the mid-1900s, when there was a more organized effort to establish models of shared decision-making.[2] As part of this effort, the rights of the patient began to be formally identified, recognizing the need to empower the patient to become a more active participant in the health-care process. The American Hospital Association developed its first version of a **Patient Bill of Rights** in 1973,[3] and many other health-care provider groups, facilities, and government health-care agencies adopted similar documents. Most patients and health-care providers now understand that patients are entitled to many rights when they are receiving health-care services.

Although there may be variations from document to document, most include the following patient rights:[1,4,5]

- To be treated with respect and dignity in a nondiscriminatory manner
- To receive safe, appropriate care
- To have procedures explained in understandable language
- To know the identity of their health-care providers
- To have some type of choice in who is providing their care
- To refuse treatment or to receive a second opinion
- To have their privacy and confidentiality maintained and protected
- To file a complaint or grievance

The APTA has also delineated the rights of patients receiving physical therapy services in the position titled "Access to, Admission to and Patient Rights Within Physical Therapy."[6]

Access to, Admission to and Patient Rights Within Physical Therapy (HOD P06-14-06-05)

In providing physical therapy services, the physical therapist is accountable first and foremost to the individual receiving physical therapy. The physical therapist is also accountable for abiding by professional standards and ethics and the laws governing the practice of physical therapy in the jurisdiction where the service is rendered. The physical therapist shall ensure services regardless of race, creed, color, gender, gender identity, gender expression, age, national or ethnic origin, sexual orientation, disability, or health status. The physical therapist respects the rights of individuals referred or admitted to the physical therapy service. The individual referred or admitted to the physical therapy service has rights that include but are not limited to:

1. Selection of a physical therapist of one's own choosing to the extent that it is reasonable and possible.
2. Access to information regarding practice policies and charges for services.
3. Knowledge of the identity of the physical therapist and other personnel providing or participating in the program of care.
4. Expectation that the referral source has no financial involvement in the service. If that is not the case, knowledge of the extent of any financial involvement in the service by the referring source.

(box continues on page 100)

Access to, Admission to and Patient Rights Within Physical Therapy (HOD P06-14-06-05) (continued)

5. Involvement in the development of anticipated goals and expected outcomes, and the selection of interventions.
6. Knowledge of any substantial risks of the recommended examination and intervention.
7. Participation in decisions involving the physical therapy plan of care to the extent reasonable and possible.
8. Access to information concerning his or her condition.
9. Expectation that any discussion or consultation involving the case will be conducted discreetly and that all communications and other records pertaining to the care, including the sources of payment for treatment, will be treated as confidential.
10. Expectation of safety in the provision of services and safety in regard to the equipment and physical environment.
11. Timely information about impending discharge and continuing care requirements.
12. Refusal of physical therapy services.
13. Information regarding the practice's mechanism for the initiation, review, and resolution of patient complaints.

Reprinted with permission of the American Physical Therapy Association. Found at http://www.apta.org/Policies. Accessed August 17, 2015. This material is copyrighted, and any further reproduction or distribution requires written permission from APTA.

Challenges for Patients in Asserting Their Rights

Patients are not always the best advocates for themselves when it comes to understanding and defending their rights. Whereas the list of commonly protected rights does not seem controversial or confusing, patients respond in many ways to illness, and those responses can affect their ability to assert their rights. Some patients still see health care as functioning in the paternalistic model, and they expect the provider to make all choices for them. They may not want to be part of any decision-making, believing that the provider is the expert. Other patients may feel too sick to participate in their own care, preferring that others take over that responsibility. Some patients may not be aware that they have any rights. Even if they have been informed of their rights upon admission to a facility or during their first physical therapy visit, they may not have been in the right frame of mind (due to pain, fatigue, anxiety, medication use, etc.) to pay attention or remember what they were told. Patients who know their rights may not have faith that they have any power to fight the medical system or to direct the plan of care. They may also have family members or close friends who have differing opinions regarding what the appropriate plan of care should include, and these people may exert undue influence on the patient or may try to influence the care providers' course of action.

Whose responsibility is it to ensure that patient rights are being protected? Everyone who interacts with the patient has some level of responsibility to do so. Primary care providers, such as a physician or a PT, may have more formal initial responsibility for explaining those rights to the patient, but everyone who works in a health-care facility has some responsibility, within the scope of their individual roles, to ensure that those rights are being maintained. Even those who do not provide direct care services, such as maintenance or housekeeping staff, have an obligation to see that the patient is treated with respect and that his privacy is maintained as much as possible. In physical therapy, the protection of patient rights is reflected in how the health-care providers interact with the patient. Simple things, such as identifying oneself and one's role as a PTA, asking the patient how he chooses to be addressed, and explaining briefly what will be happening in a given day's intervention session, can make a huge difference in how the patient perceives his involvement in his own care and whether he perceives the interaction with the provider to be positive or negative.

At the beginning of an episode of care, the evaluating PT should obtain **informed consent** from the patient (or in cases in which patients cannot provide consent, from their designated representative). This is a multistep process that is often required by law and should include the following:[2]

- Explanation of the findings of the examination/evaluation, identification of the physical therapy diagnosis, and description of the interventions that will be delivered to treat that diagnosis. Included with this should be discussion of the risks, benefits, and alternatives to the interventions prescribed.
- Opportunity for the patient to ask questions about the examination/evaluation, diagnosis, prognosis, or proposed interventions.
- A formal request for permission to proceed with the plan of care.

During subsequent intervention sessions, the PT/PTA should continue to explain to the patient in advance what is scheduled for that day's interventions. It is important not only to gain consent for those interventions but also to give the patient options (as appropriate) regarding how they are delivered. For example, the PTA might give a patient a choice of performing balance drills prior to performing strengthening exercises or a choice of receiving therapy at bedside instead of in the therapy department. Giving him some say in the intervention session can lead to the patient feeling more respected by and included in the therapy team.

FOR REFLECTION

- Imagine that you are walking into a patient's room to deliver physical therapy services. When you introduce yourself, the patient states, "I don't feel well. I don't want to do any physical therapy today." Would you try to talk him into participating, even though he has already expressed a desire not to participate? Defend your answer.

HIPAA

One of the most important rights afforded to patients is the right to privacy and confidentiality. It is also one of the rights most easily (though often unintentionally) compromised. Providers may communicate about their patients to people uninvolved with the patient's care (for example, telling a friend about a specific patient) or in a way that allows others not involved to have access to the information (such as discussing a patient with coworkers in an elevator or in the facility's cafeteria). The advances in electronic telecommunication (voice mail, faxes, e-mail, etc.) have also increased the possibility that private health-care information can be shared inadvertently with others who have no right to know it. To protect the rights of privacy and confidentiality better, the federal government passed the **Health Insurance Portability and Accountability Act (HIPAA)** in 1996. Part of this act mandated that providers develop standard procedures for ensuring that confidential patient information (including electronically shared information) remains secure and that patients are aware of their rights regarding privacy of information.[7] Generally, all employees are now required to participate in training on their facility's procedures for following HIPAA guidelines at the time of their hiring and at regularly scheduled intervals throughout their employment. Students in health-care programs are usually required to have some general HIPAA training at their academic institution prior to being sent out on clinical experiences and then may receive more facility-specific training at a given site. Much of this training will include directives on:

- How to keep confidential patient information private.
- How to determine which employees of a facility should be allowed to have access to confidential information, often generalized as consisting of only those with a "need to know" about the patient depending on the specifics of a patient's situation.
- Appropriate ways of using electronic telecommunication equipment for transmitting patient information and ensuring that it stays secure.
- Strategies for avoiding unintentional sharing of information.

Patient Reactions to Illness and Injury: Psychosocial Factors That Affect the Patient-PTA Relationship

As stated, most health-care providers now understand that it is inappropriate (and often detrimental to success) if the patient is a passive recipient of medical care. Many patient bill of rights documents now include lists of patients' responsibilities in taking an active role in their plan of care to ensure that patients do their best to promote positive outcomes.[2] However, patients often have difficulty fulfilling these responsibilities. This can be challenging or frustrating to providers. Thinking about the various ways that people respond to illness and injury may enhance understanding of why this occurs.

FOR REFLECTION
FOR REFLECTION

■ Think about how you have acted in the past when you have been ill with a cold or the flu. Are you someone who wants others to take care of you while you are sick, or do you prefer that people just leave you alone until you get better? Do you go to bed (or to your physician) at the first sign of illness, or do you "tough it out" until you are too sick to continue with normal activities? Carry these thoughts over to when you are working with patients. How could their different responses to illness or injury affect their participation in a therapy program?

People react to injury and illness in many ways. Their reactions may differ based on their individual personality type (as discussed in the For Reflection box), their potential for recovery or improvement, their support systems, their belief systems, and their views on how the injury or illness will affect their life. Many patients go through a grieving process, similar to what one goes through when affected by the loss of a loved one, especially if the nature of the diagnosis is likely to leave the patient with permanent physical or lifestyle changes. Many models describe the processes that patients may go through in dealing with a loss. One well-known model of the **stages of grief,** as described by Kübler-Ross, includes the following:[8]

- Denial
- Anger
- Bargaining
- Depression
- Acceptance

Other emotional reactions may include fear (of pain, of changes in their societal role, of loss of independence, and so on), having a negative body image (especially with a disfiguring illness or injury), feeling sorry for oneself, and a feeling of loss of all control. Although all of these reactions are normal responses to disability, they can interfere with a patient's ability to participate fully in his rehabilitation, sometimes more than the illness or injury itself.[9] To deal with these emotions, patients may employ various coping strategies, which can either be positive (for example, keeping a journal or encouraging other patients during their therapy sessions) or negative (such as refusing to attend therapy or demonstrating inappropriate sexual behavior). When a patient's inability to cope with the reality of his medical situation affects his progress, the PTA should address the issue with the supervising PT. To best serve the patient, providers may discuss the situation with other members of the health-care team who have expertise in psychosocial issues, such as a psychologist, psychiatrist, social worker, or chaplain.

The Provider's Response to the Patient's Psychosocial Needs

Patients respond differently to the events occurring in their lives, and reactions and responses to each patient need to be different, based on that patient's needs. Although the patient may feel sorry for himself, it is not in his best interests if the health-care providers feel sorry for him, too. Clinicians have a responsibility to help patients develop a sense of hope, but patients may have difficulty feeling hopeful if they sense that their care providers feel sorry for them or pity them, as these emotions have a more negative connotation. Patients respond better when their providers demonstrate a sense of **empathy.**

Developing empathy is described by Davis as a process in which providers go beyond just being able to put themselves in their patients' situations to being able to perceive the patient's frame of reference. They then use that insight to connect more effectively with the patient.[10] The clinician must be careful while attempting to demonstrate empathetic behavior that he does not come across as insincere. For example, saying to a patient, "I know how you must be feeling," no matter how well-intentioned, may provoke an angry response such as, "How could you know what I am feeling? You have never experienced this!" The PTA has now lost credibility in the eyes of the patient. A better strategy may be to lead with the statement, "I haven't been in your position, but I imagine that if I were, I might be feeling …" or just to have the patient state what he is experiencing.

Patients also benefit from a sense of **empowerment.** Empowerment is the process of enabling patients to take an active leadership role in their health-care decisions.[1] This can be done in part by educating patients about their options and responsibilities and engaging them in the process of intervention selection, goal setting, and problem-solving.[11] Conscious use of language that puts the patient first ("the patient who has sustained a cerebrovascular accident [CVA]" instead of "the CVA patient" or worse yet, "the CVA") or that has a less negative connotation ("a patient who has cancer" instead of "a *victim* of cancer" or "a patient *suffering* from cancer") can subtly assist with promoting empowerment.[9,10]

Advocacy and Accountability

Advocacy is defined as the process of asserting oneself to represent the needs of a particular group or individual.[1] In health care, the patients are the group whose needs should be kept in mind and be considered above all others' needs. This advocacy may lead to the PTA taking a proactive role in interacting with other health-care providers, with family members, or with other groups within the health-care system who have their own opinions of how to best advocate for the patient's needs.

Patients may have difficulty in asserting their rights and may require the assistance of the PTA to make sure their voices are heard. For example, a patient in acute care may mention that he refused to take a shower that morning because the nursing assistant who offered the shower was of the opposite sex. Knowing that the patient has the right, when possible, to have a provider of his choosing, the PTA could discuss the patient's reasons for refusal with the nursing staff in an attempt to make that arrangement.

A patient may also have difficulty in advocating for himself within the context of his own family. For example, it is not unusual for children of an aging family member, especially if they believe that the patient is demonstrating signs of cognitive decline, to take a more assertive role in speaking for or making decisions for the patient without necessarily having the authority to do so. This may also involve withholding information from the patient. A PTA, in working with a patient who has been recently diagnosed with terminal cancer, may learn from the patient's family that they have not shared the true prognosis of the disease with the patient, telling him that he will make a full recovery. The PTA can serve as an advocate for the patient's right to know about his diagnosis by sharing this information with the supervising PT, a social worker, or other health-care providers who can best determine if the patient's rights are being violated.

In addition to advocating for individual patients, a PTA might serve in an advocacy role as part of a larger group, such as a professional organization or place of employment.[1] Working with a group, such as the APTA, gives individual PTs and PTAs more resources (financial, organizational, personnel) to create a stronger voice in advocating for their group's needs. Most of these groups exist, at least in part, to serve the needs of patients. The APTA's "Professionalism in Physical Therapy: Core Values" identifies "advocating for the health and wellness needs of society" as well as for "changes in laws, regulations, standards and guidelines that affect physical therapist service provision" as part of the member's social responsibility role.[12] Sometimes advocacy groups can work together, such as when the APTA has worked with the American Occupational Therapy Association and the American Speech-Language-Hearing Association to challenge Medicare regulations.

PTAs may also find that their advocacy role can be enhanced through involvement outside the health-care arena, either individually or as a member of other advocacy groups. Being active politically, regardless of a particular party, provides an opportunity to stand up for a variety of patient needs. Participating in nonpolitical activism groups, such as neighborhood associations, environmental groups, and school organizations, may also allow advocacy for the needs of patients beyond health care. This also has the additional benefit of helping the PTA to develop leadership traits, a concept that is addressed in Chapter 12.

FOR REFLECTION
FOR REFLECTION

- Being an advocate sometimes means having to defend your convictions to people in authority. Do you have the type of personality to be comfortable doing this? Why or why not? If not, what can you do to develop that ability?

Another core value that patients expect to see demonstrated by their caregivers is **accountability.** Being accountable is doing what one says one will do. This can be done generally, such as upholding legal and ethical obligations as identified in Chapters 5 and 10, and can be demonstrated specifically, such as seeing the patient on time, following through on promises (such as delivering a request for more pain medication to the patient's nurse), or assisting the patient with a toilet transfer rather than telling the patient to call for the nursing assistant. Accountability is also reflected in the PTA's ability to document accurately and appropriately (see Chapter 8).

Conflicts Between the PTA'S Personal and Professional Values

In the process of empowering patients to advocate for themselves, providers sometimes have difficulty accepting a patient's choice that differs from what the health-care provider believes is the "right" choice, such as when a patient refuses to attend physical therapy sessions. Additionally, it can be challenging when the patient demonstrates lifestyle choices or behaviors that a provider knows to be detrimental (such as smoking cigarettes) or in opposition to one's own morals and values (such as a patient who engages in criminal activity). Health-care providers are the persons of "power," the ones with the most control, in the patient-provider relationship. Along with this power comes the obligation to ensure that the provider's own values or biases do not interfere with the patient's ability to make choices, even if those choices potentially interfere with the patient's likelihood of demonstrating progress in rehabilitation. The Standards of Ethical Conduct for the Physical Therapist Assistant (see Chapter 5) require PTAs to treat all patients in a nonjudgmental manner, regardless of whether the PTA agrees with their actions or value systems. Part of empowering the patient requires being able to let go of the paternalistic view that providers know what is best.[11]

The Role of Communication in the Patient-PTA Relationship

Developing a sense of empowerment is one example of how the core value of compassion/caring is demonstrated in day-to-day physical therapist practice.[12] It is also demonstrated by how we communicate with the patient. The term **rapport** is often used to describe the sense of connection between providers and their clients. Rapport is described as a relationship of mutual trust and understanding,[1,13] and it is developed only when providers can effectively communicate that sense of caring to the patient. Chapter 3 discusses the communication strategies that are essential for the success of the PT/PTA team. Similarly, effective communication is also the key to building a successful patient-PTA relationship. Developing expertise in patient communication is both an art and a skill, and entire texts have been devoted to improving awareness and abilities in this area. This discussion is designed to provide an overview of the key concepts to be considered when developing communication skills. For additional strategies and information, see the references at the end of this chapter.

Communication: More Than Talking

Words are only a small component of how people communicate with each other. The manner in which the words are delivered, the nonverbal messages that are demonstrated while words are being spoken, and the way in which one listens to the words of others are all components of communication, and in many ways they may be more important to comprehension of the message than the words themselves.

FOR REFLECTION

- Have you ever sent someone an e-mail or a text message that was misinterpreted? Think about why the message did not come across as you intended. If you had spoken the words to the other person, what might have occurred that would have prevented the words from being misunderstood?

Most people have a preferred style of communicating with others. These styles are often related to one's personality, and it is even more likely that the styles developed as a result of the environment or culture in which one was raised.[14] It is the PTA's responsibility to recognize that his style of communication may differ from that of the patient and then to alter his methods as appropriate to best meet the patient's needs to make the best possible connection. The following section outlines the elements that should be taken into consideration when developing verbal and nonverbal communication skills.

Verbal Elements of Communication

Introductions and Titles

The PTA should always introduce himself and identify himself as a PTA. He should then verify the patient's identity ("You are Mr. Robert Harris, correct?") and then ask him how he prefers to be addressed (Mr. Harris, Robert, Bob, and so on). For patients with cognitive deficits or those who are seen irregularly or in a setting such as acute care where they are being exposed to a number of providers, the PTA should reintroduce himself at the start of every intervention session unless he is sure that the patient remembers him.

Clarity and Directness

People have different styles in how they deliver the content of their verbal messages. Some are very direct and come to a point immediately, whereas others will talk about other subjects before getting to the main subject of a conversation. The PTA must use language that is clear and concise to promote understanding and to be efficient. The rapid pace of today's health-care environment encourages this direct style of communication, but some patients may be offended if the provider delivers information in a straightforward manner that is perceived to be impersonal or rushed.

The patient who is resistant to physical therapy may respond better to an approach that is more subtle. The PTA may need to spend a few moments chatting about seemingly irrelevant information to establish a rapport with the patient before asking him to attend physical therapy or perform a given task.

Tone, Volume, and Speed

The PTA should work to ensure that his words are delivered in such a way that they are easily heard and understood. This includes using a tone that reflects warmth yet is professional, and one that does not imply superiority or condescension (this is occasionally seen in caregivers who work with older adults or those with cognitive impairments). The PTA must also vary the volume or pitch of his voice, dependent on the patient's hearing needs, and should use a speed of delivery that allows for variations in patient processing. Silence can be also used as a tool to allow the patient time to assimilate information.

Language Appropriate for the Patient's Level of Understanding

The PTA's choice of vocabulary may vary depending on the age and background of the person. Unless the patient has a health-care background, the use of medical terminology should be avoided or clearly defined. Patients may not feel comfortable stating that they do not understand a term used by the PTA. In response to a PTA's question that contains unfamiliar medical jargon, the patient might try to guess at the content, resulting in a potentially inappropriate or inaccurate response.

Quantity of Information Given

The PTA should monitor the amount of information given to the patient at any one time, allowing for processing time, especially in situations in which cognitive impairment is involved. What may seem like routine, commonly known information to health-care providers may be new information for the patient and could be overwhelming if given in large amounts.

Checking for Comprehension

It is always a good idea to make sure that the patient understands any directions or instructions that have been given to him by the PTA. Having the patient repeat the directions is one way to check for comprehension. This is especially true if there is any type of cognitive, hearing, or language barrier (issues related to differences in language are addressed later in this chapter). Make sure that the patient knows his intelligence is not being questioned; the focus should be on whether the PTA used an appropriate amount of clarity and detail in giving the initial instruction.

Use of Questions

In addition to using questions to ensure comprehension, the PTA should also use them to obtain information from the patient or others involved in his care. **Open-ended questions** (those that require the patient to give more than a "yes/no" or one-word answer) will encourage the patient to share more information, enabling the PTA to gain a more complete picture of the patient's history and concerns. This, in turn, can also lead to the patient feeling more empowered, because he senses that his opinions and input are valued and necessary.[11]

Use of Humor

The use of humor, while at times effective in reducing the stress of a situation, can also be risky. What one person considers humorous can often be offensive to another. In addition, the effect of a serious illness or perceived medical crisis may make a patient more sensitive to humor or alter a patient's ability to respond to it. The PTA can never be sure that a patient will interpret the use of humor in the manner in which it was intended; therefore, it is best to err on the side of caution, at least until the PTA has a sense of the patient's affect and personality. A patient who uses humor in his conversation may be more open to the use of it by the provider, but again, the PTA must maintain a professional manner at all times. If a patient uses humor that is inappropriate or offensive to the PTA, the PTA may choose to ignore it, redirect the patient, or inform the patient (using a professional tone and manner) that the use of humor was not appropriate.

FOR REFLECTION

- Have you ever been around someone who told a joke that offended you? How did you respond? Later, did you wish you had responded differently? Why can it be challenging to tell someone that something he said was inappropriate?

Nonverbal Elements of Communication

Nonverbal components of language often have a greater effect on how messages are interpreted than do the words.[11,13] The way in which nonverbal messages are interpreted can be culturally dependent or influenced by the mind-set of the person being addressed.[14] The PTA should observe the patient's use of nonverbal communication while monitoring one's own to ensure that it matches the verbal message. Following the patient's lead in the use of nonverbal communication is a strategy often used to connect more effectively on this level.[11] Considerations for appropriate nonverbal communication are discussed next.

Facial Expressions and Body Language

Facial expressions and body language communicate with others even before words are spoken. When entering a patient's room, what first impression does the PTA give the patient? Does the PTA appear happy to be at work and confident in his abilities, or does he appear hurried and disorganized? First impressions are often difficult to erase. Furthermore, when body language and spoken words contradict each other, the listener is more likely to perceive the body language as being more accurate.[9,11] The PTA needs to be aware of what message his expressions and body language could be giving to patients. When a patient asks for assistance with a task, does the PTA roll his eyes while providing that assistance? If so, the patient may interpret that to mean the PTA thinks the patient is not trying hard enough, when the PTA might actually have been frustrated with his own inability to recognize that the patient required assistance. Body language that is consistent with the words spoken and that encourages the patient to be open with his thoughts and concerns will facilitate a better connection between the patient and the PTA.

Eye Contact

For those raised in the dominant U.S. culture, a lack of direct eye contact may be interpreted as a lack of interest or a sign of poor self-confidence. However, those raised in other cultures may consider direct eye contact to be disrespectful or offensive. The PTA needs to remember that his preference for eye contact may not match that of the patient. If attempting to make direct eye contact, the PTA should also remember that his body's position while looking at the patient can also influence the interpretation of his words. For a patient in a wheelchair, having to look up at a PTA who is standing while talking may not only cause the patient to feel that he is in an inferior position but may also cause physical discomfort in the neck or back. The PTA should try to maintain a level eye position with the patient when direct eye contact is being used.

Personal Space and Touch

There are wide variations in how close people choose to be to each other or how much physical contact they use while speaking. If a patient has mobility challenges, he may not be able to control how closely he is positioned to others or the level of physical contact he has with them (either too much or too little). The PTA needs to be sensitive to the patient's personal space requirements and tolerance for touch, always erring on the side of caution and being conservative in his sense of the patient's comfort zones. Even though touch is used to express caring and is thought to promote healing, it can also be easily misinterpreted.[11] Touching patients is often a necessary component of physical therapy intervention. It is essential that any touch, especially that which the patient cannot see or could be misinterpreted as having a sexual connotation (such as having to stabilize a patient's ischial tuberosity while performing a hip flexor stretch), be explained and permission to touch first obtained.

Physical Appearance of the Provider

Patients (and clinicians) of different ages, cultures, and socioeconomic status may have very different interpretations of what "professional appearance" entails. In addition, what is appropriate attire or appearance in one setting may not be appropriate in another. For example, an acute care setting might require the use of laboratory coats, but clients in an assisted living setting may prefer that their providers wear street clothes because of the residential nature of that setting. In any setting, the physical appearance of the PTA should not distract the patient from focusing on his physical therapy interventions. For example, if a PTA's hair is always falling in front of his eyes and he is constantly pushing it back, the patient may become focused on watching this and not on the directions the PTA is providing. Clothing that is too tight or too revealing may also distract patients and may result in the PTA being labeled as unprofessional, regardless of the quality of the care provided.

Attitude and Focus

Students and new graduates in particular may have difficulty not showing stress in front of a patient, but it is extremely important that the provider's words reflect an aura of confidence and professionalism. The PTA should work at appearing at ease, not nervous or rushed, with his full concentration on that particular patient. Each person with whom the PTA interacts should feel that he is the sole object of the PTA's focus at that time. This may be difficult to do in a physical environment in which the PTA is frequently being interrupted or distracted. The patient's attention likewise may become diverted by other activity or noise in the room. Working with patients in a room as free of distractions as possible may help both parties keep focused on their interaction.

Listening Skills

In order for the patient-PTA relationship to be most effective, the PTA must also develop strong listening skills. Listening is much more than just hearing. Most of us can probably think of times when we talked to someone at length but ended the conversation feeling as if the other person really did not hear what we were trying to say.

FOR REFLECTION

- Think about someone who is a good listener. What does that person do to make you know that you are being heard? How does knowing that you are being heard make you feel?

Without feedback from the person to whom you are listening, there is no way to be sure you are interpreting the message correctly. A strategy used to ensure comprehension is **active listening.** This is especially effective if the speaker seems to be having difficulty expressing himself. Active listening consists of three components that are used to interpret the speaker's message instead of simply reacting to it.[10]

- **Restatement:** After the speaker says something, the listener says it back to him, often in the form of a question, without adding any interpretation at this point.
  Patient: "I'm not going to therapy today! I hate exercising!"
  PTA: "You don't want to go to physical therapy today?"
- **Reflection:** The listener then not only comments on the content of what the speaker says but also adds his interpretation of what was meant by the words.
  PTA: "You don't like exercising. The exercises must be very difficult."
- **Clarification:** The listener then gives the speaker the opportunity to correct his interpretation of the speaker's words.
  PTA: "Is that what you don't like about physical therapy?"

This final component is critical, especially if the listener is unsure of his interpretation; if the interpretation is incorrect, the speaker will continue to feel that he is not being heard.

The Influence of Culture on Communication

Chapter 7 addresses how culture means much more than country of origin or language spoken. Differences related to these two components of culture can have a particular influence on the effectiveness of patient-PTA communication. This chapter has already addressed how the environment in which a patient has been raised can influence the preferred style of communication. The additional challenges involved when two people speak different languages are obvious. Some ways of dealing with these challenges are more effective than others. For purposes of addressing language issues in this section, it is assumed that English is the primary language used when delivering physical therapy services.

If there is any question about whether a patient is effectively able to communicate because of a difference in language, an interpreter should be used. Even if the patient appears to speak English effectively enough to respond to the PTA, he may not comprehend everything he is told. The interpreter should be a formally trained health-care interpreter or a neutral party (such as a person in the department who speaks that language) who will deliver the message to the patient exactly as it has been spoken. Family members may not always understand the medical jargon or may change the message if they disagree with what the provider is saying. An example of this might be a family member who believes the PTA is not making the patient work hard enough and tells the patient to do more repetitions of an exercise than the PTA really said. Conversely, patients may not be comfortable sharing all of their concerns in front of family members (for example, a woman having pain during sexual activity may not be comfortable having her teenage son interpret that message for her). At times, there may be no option other than a family member. If this is the case, the PTA should pay extra attention to the patient's facial expressions, body language, and the length of the message as stated by the patient as compared with the length of the message in translation to help ensure that messages are being communicated accurately.

Accents and dialects can also interfere with effectively conveying a message. The PTA must remember that what is considered an accent to one person may not be considered an accent to others. When working with a patient whose message is not clear because of an accent, it may be awkward to have to ask him to repeat himself multiple times. However, this is preferred over pretending to understand what the patient said. Even if that which is not understood is not critical to the care of the patient, the patient is likely to know, based on the PTA's response (or lack of response), that his message was not understood, and this may affect his willingness to attempt further communication. Asking the patient to speak slowly or to rephrase the statement that was not understood may enhance the provider's ability to comprehend it. If the PTA is the person with the accent, he must acknowledge this to the patient, and must stress the importance of letting the PTA know when his message is not being understood. Many patients are reluctant to tell providers they do not understand something told to them (even without language barriers) and may be even more hesitant to do so when an accent is involved for fear of offending the speaker. By proactively acknowledging the potential for communication breakdown due to an accent, the PTA is giving the patient permission to ask more questions without fear of offending.

Strategies to Improve Communication in Times of Breakdown

There will be times when effective communication with the patient breaks down. As stated previously, the PTA is the person with the most power in the patient-PTA relationship and thus must take the initiative to do everything possible to restore the lines of communication. If the PTA is able to accept at least a portion of responsibility for the problems that have occurred, demonstrate a willingness to improve the lines of communication, and suggest strategies to avoid future problems, then the other person involved is more likely to do the same and the potential for improvement is greater.

When discussing conflicts, not only with patients but also with classmates, clinical instructors, or supervisors, keep emotions regarding the situation in check and keep the conversation to the facts about what occurred. This can be difficult, as conflict usually creates some type of internal tension that affects our emotional state.[9] The technique of using **"I" messages,** such as "I felt really frustrated when I was trying to explain the exercises," instead of the "you" message of "You weren't listening to me very well," is a well-known strategy for discussing perceptions of conflict with the other person.[10] It is effective in that it becomes difficult for the other individual to argue with the factual validity of the first "I" message, as the patient cannot know how the PTA feels. However, if the second statement is used, the patient is likely to reply defensively, "Yes, I was!" and respond back with a "you" message of his own.

Another strategy involves avoiding use of the terms "never" and "always." The absolute nature of those words often leads someone to respond defensively, as it is unlikely that someone *always* or *never* does something in a certain way. Being more accurate and objective in one's statement (i.e., "You have been late two times this week" rather than "You are always late to your therapy appointments") is more likely to keep the conflict related to the facts of the situation.

In the long run, the patient's functional goals are the ultimate outcome to be considered. The definitive obligation of any health-care provider is to the patient, and the PTA, like any other provider, must recognize when communication issues are interfering with the patient's ability to demonstrate progress. When a PTA is involved in scenarios involving conflict, it is essential to involve the supervising PT, both as a somewhat neutral third party and as the person who has ultimate responsibility for the patient. Sometimes a patient may need to be reassigned to someone else's schedule so that he has the opportunity to develop a better connection with his provider, promoting the best possible outcomes. However, this is not always feasible, and it can be a blow to any PTA's confidence. Developing the ability to connect with any patient, regardless of his personality, life choices, or differing communication styles, will minimize the likelihood that this will occur.

SUMMARY

The ability to connect with patients through the development of strong interpersonal communication skills is essential to success of the patient-PTA relationship. In addition to using effective communication strategies, other responsibilities that the PTA has within this relationship include helping to ensure that the patient's rights are protected, advocating for the patient's needs, and empowering the patient to actively take a lead role in the rehabilitation process.

REFERENCES

1. Venes D, ed. *Taber's Encyclopedic Medical Dictionary.* 22nd ed. Philadelphia, PA: FA Davis; 2013.
2. Scott RW. *Foundations of Physical Therapy.* New York, NY: McGraw-Hill; 2002:484.
3. Virginia Health Information. Changes in hospital care: The patient's bill of rights. http://www.vhi.org/hguide_patientbill.asp. Updated 2015. Accessed August 17, 2015.
4. American Medical Association. Opinion 10.01: fundamental elements of the patient-physician relationship. http://www.ama-assn.org/ama/pub/physician-resources/medical-ethics/code-medical-ethics/opinion1001.shtml. Updated 1993. Accessed August 17, 2015.
5. Association of American Physicians and Surgeons. Patients' bill of rights. http://www.aapsonline.org/patients/billrts.htm. Updated 1995. Accessed August 17, 2015.
6. American Physical Therapy Association. Access to, admission to and patient/client rights within physical therapy (HOD P06-14-06-05). http://www.apta.org/uploadedFiles/APTAorg/About_Us/Policies/Practice/AccessAdmissionPatient ClientRights.pdf. Updated 2014. Accessed August 17, 2015.

7. US Department of Health and Human Services. Health information privacy. http://www.hhs.gov/ocr/privacy/. Updated 2015. Accessed August 17, 2015.

8. Kübler-Ross E. *On Death and Dying: What the Dying Have to Teach Doctors, Nurses, Clergy and Their Own Families.* New York, NY: Scribner; 2003:286.

9. Drench ME, Noonan AC, Sharby N, Ventura SH. *Psychosocial Aspects of Health Care.* 2nd ed. Upper Saddle River, NJ: Pearson Prentice Hall; 2007:364.

10. Davis CM. *Patient Practitioner Interaction: An Experiential Manual for Developing the Art of Health Care.* 5th ed. Thorofare, NJ: SLACK; 2011:274. http://www.loc.gov/catdir/toc/ ecip0518/2005022063.html.

11. Arnold EC, Boggs KU. *Interpersonal Relationships: Professional Communication Skills for Nurses.* 6th ed. St. Louis, MO: Saunders Elsevier; 2011:547.

12. American Physical Therapy Association. Professionalism in physical therapy: core values (BOD P05-04-02-03). http://www.apta.org/uploadedFiles/APTAorg/About_Us/Policies/Judicial_Legal/ProfessionalismCoreValues.pdf. Updated 2012. Accessed August 10, 2015.

13. Mueller M. *Communication From the Inside Out: Strategies for the Engaged Professional.* Philadelphia, PA: FA Davis; 2010:370.

14. Lattanzi JB, Purnell LD. *Developing Cultural Competence in Physical Therapy Practice.* Philadelphia, PA: FA Davis; 2006:417.

Name _____

REVIEW

1. List the eight rights that are generally protected in patient rights documents.

_____

_____

_____

_____

_____

_____

_____

_____

2. Give examples of how you could use three different verbal techniques to facilitate effective communication with patients.

_____

_____

_____

_____

3. Give examples of how you could use three different nonverbal techniques to facilitate effective communication with patients.

_____

_____

_____

_____

(questions continue on page 118)

Application

1. You are performing your documentation at the nursing station of a skilled nursing facility. A physician and nurse practitioner are performing rounds at the facility today, but while they are standing by the nursing station, they begin to talk to each other about the patients they saw yesterday at another facility. They begin laughing about the inappropriate behavior of residents with cognitive issues, and the physician mentions one resident by name. The person they are discussing is a relative of yours, and you are disturbed by the comments they are making about him.

   A. What rights (if any) are being violated in this situation?

   _____

   _____

   _____

   _____

   B. Would you address your concerns with the physician and nurse practitioner? Is there anyone else with whom you would discuss this? Write down what you might say.

   _____

   _____

   _____

   _____

2. Review the scenario at the beginning of this chapter. Mr. Erickson and his daughter have now arrived for his intervention session. You notice that when you ask Mr. Erickson a question, the daughter frequently interrupts him during his response or disagrees with what he says. You are concerned that Mr. Erickson is not being given the opportunity to speak for himself. In the space below, write down what you might say to his daughter to address your concerns.

   _____

   _____

   _____

   _____

3. Using the active listening techniques, respond to the following patient statement:

"Why should I go to therapy? I'm not getting better! I'm going to have to stay here forever!"

Restatement: _____

Reflection: _____

Clarification: _____

4. Correct the following statements a PTA might make to others so that they are delivered in a manner that facilitates more effective communication:

To a patient: "You're not doing your exercises at home!"

_____

_____

_____

_____

To a colleague: "You aren't listening to me!"

_____

_____

_____

_____

To your supervisor: "I always have to work late!"

_____

_____

_____

_____

7

The Impact of Culture and Spirituality on the Delivery of Physical Therapy Interventions

CHAPTER OBJECTIVES

After reading the chapter, the reader will be able to:

- Identify trends in the diversity of the U.S. population and the physical therapy profession.
- Compare and contrast cultural awareness, cultural competency, and cultural proficiency.
- Give examples of the elements that might define an individual's culture.
- Describe how an individual's culture, values, and biases are developed.
- Discuss the utilization of self-awareness and reflection as a means of understanding personal values and biases.
- Discuss how issues of privilege and power differentials contribute to the development of disparities in the U.S. health-care system.
- Describe the benefits of supporting the client's belief system.
- Recognize how the use of cultural generalizations must be balanced with individual interaction to avoid stereotyping.
- Give examples of how to provide culturally appropriate services.
- Define spirituality as a component of culture.
- Compare and contrast spirituality and religion.
- Recognize spirituality's effect on health, illness, and end-of-life issues.
- Identify ways to develop comfort and capability in dealing with issues of culture and spirituality.

KEY TERMS AND CONCEPTS

- Culture
- Cultural pre-competence/competence/proficiency
- Covert bias
- Service learning
- Privilege
- Health-care disparities
- Overt/covert norms
- Spirituality

Tyrell is a newly graduated physical therapist assistant (PTA) working in an acute care setting. Today he is seeing all his patients at bedside. When he goes into the room of his first patient, a woman who has sustained a cerebrovascular accident, he is surprised to find that she has a number of visitors who appear to have been there all night. Tyrell tells the patient that it is time for her therapy session and asks everyone to leave the room. One man identifies himself as the patient's husband and states, "It's too early for therapy. She has been awake most of the night and doesn't feel well. I don't think she should have physical therapy right now until she's feeling better." Tyrell asks the patient, "What do you think?" but the patient only looks up at her husband and remains silent. Tyrell says, "Let's give it a try" and again asks the visitors to leave. The patient's husband becomes angry and says, "Why do we have to leave? What are you going to do to her?" The patient also becomes agitated, and, seeing this, the husband says, "Now you've upset her. She can't do therapy now. You will have to come back later."

QUESTIONS TO CONSIDER

Did Tyrell need to ask the family to leave? What are some valid reasons for his having done so? Did asking the family to leave play a role in the patient's willingness to participate in the therapy session? Are there factors other than the patient's tolerance for therapy that might be affecting the family's willingness to let her participate? Why is the patient not speaking for herself?

Who Are You?

Take a moment to think about how you would respond to this question: Who are you? Write down a few of the descriptors you would use. Now, if possible, share your responses with someone else who has done the same thing. Did you use descriptors that were similar, or did the other person define herself in a way that you did not consider? This chapter discusses why these similarities or differences may have occurred.

Was it uncomfortable for you to discuss the above with someone else? If so, you are not alone. Issues related to culture, as a reflection of who people are, are often extremely personal and difficult to discuss. However, if issues of culture are not discussed, certain assumptions may be made about who someone is, how that person identifies herself, or whether certain aspects of her cultural identity are more important to her than others. This chapter also discusses the concepts of cultural generalizations and stereotypes.

What Is Culture?

Culture is a multifaceted term that has been defined in many ways, but it generally refers to the beliefs, values, and norms that people use to identify who they are and how to interact with others.[1] Padilla and Brown consider culture an individualized "lens" through which people view themselves, each other, and society as a whole.[2] A few components of what one identifies as one's culture may be shaped by genetics, but it is mostly influenced by one's upbringing and individual life experiences. A person's expectations in beliefs and behaviors are developed in an unconscious process.[3] Some biological cultural components are fixed or "static," but many aspects of culture are fluid, and their presence or relevance change throughout one's life.

It is important to be able to recognize one's own cultural beliefs and practices because they influence interactions with others. Sometimes, what one perceives to be happening in a situation is different from what might be occurring from another's point of view.

FOR REFLECTION

- In the initial scenario, the patient's husband spoke, and the patient did not. What was your initial interpretation of the reason this occurred? Are there other possible explanations for why this occurred?

Components of Cultural Diversity

As the population of the United States has grown larger, it has become increasingly more diverse. Most people associate the term "diversity" with the differences between individuals or groups of individuals. It is a term that has become commonly associated with ethnic or racial differences. However, it is important to recognize that race and ethnicity are only two components of the cultural diversity that can occur between individuals or groups. Some types of diversity may seem to be readily apparent, but other types may not be as discernible or may be kept "hidden." The analogy of an iceberg is often used in describing how most cultural components are "under water," with the visible part, the "tip," being only a small portion of what is present. Some components of diversity are relatively fixed (often called primary cultural characteristics), whereas others can be changed, depending on a person's life circumstances and desires (referred to as secondary characteristics).[4] Age, gender, sexual orientation, religious beliefs, socioeconomic status, political views, and physical appearance (e.g., hair color, weight, style of dress) are some of the other primary and secondary components that can contribute to cultural diversity. These factors can drive how an individual sees herself in relation to the rest of society and can shape how that person views her interactions with others. This chapter does not discuss all these types of differences but assumes that all of them and more are considered components of cultural diversity.

FOR REFLECTION

FOR REFLECTION

- List as many components of culture as you can, including the ones already listed. Of this list, which ones are visible, and which are hidden? Which are fixed (or primary) components, and which are changeable (secondary)? If possible, compare your list with that of someone else. Did you classify all components into the same categories? If not, discuss your rationales for the differences in classification.

Recognizing that race and ethnicity are only two components of culture, reviewing data about the ethnic makeup of the U.S. population is still useful, given how often diversity is connected to ethnicity. Whereas the dominant racial classification continues to include those who identify themselves racially as "white only," the 2010 U.S. Census found that 27.6 percent of the population identified themselves as being some other race than "white only," an increase of 2.7 percent from the 2000 census. All racial groups in the 2010 census showed a greater percentage of growth than the white-only group, with those identifying their race as "Asian" showing the largest percentage of increase. In the 2010 census, over 9 million people (about 3 percent of the total) identified themselves as being of more than one race. The 2010 census did not use "Hispanic" as a racial category, stating its belief that those of Hispanic background may identify with any race, but those who identified themselves as being of Hispanic ethnicity in the 2010 census increased by 3.8 percent.[5] More and more people are identifying themselves as multiracial or of multiple ethnic backgrounds, with race being used less and less to define someone. Given all of these changes, it is difficult and risky to make assumptions about anyone's racial or ethnic identification based solely on appearance.[6]

Diversity in Physical Therapy

The ethnic diversity of the population is mirrored in the diversity of those becoming health-care workers, although certain health-care professions have become more ethnically diverse than others. Again, the PTA must remember that the race or ethnicity with which one identifies may or may not be easily discernible to others. In physical therapy, the self-identified descriptors of those entering the field continue to be predominantly female and white. Although current data show that the enrollment of minority students in both PT and PTA programs is around 20 percent,[7,8] the overall representation of non-whites currently in the profession is under 10 percent. Historically, the average age of those becoming PTAs has tended to be somewhat higher than the average age of those currently entering doctor of physical therapy programs.[9]

The American Physical Therapy Association (APTA) has developed a number of initiatives designed to help promote more ethnic diversity within physical therapy. The APTA's Committee on Cultural Competence has developed an operational plan that identifies strategies for changing the demographics of those entering PT and PTA programs (and of those becoming APTA members) to accurately "reflect the changing demographics of U.S. society."[10] In 1988, the APTA created the Minority Scholarship Fund. Aided by fund-raising events, the Minority Scholarship Fund has issued hundreds of thousands of dollars' worth of scholarships to students of color and diverse ethnic backgrounds.[11]

The Spectrum of Cultural Sensitivity

Expertise in dealing with issues of culture has frequently been referred to as being developed on a continuum; a person becomes more and more conscious of the issues, usually by way of more exposure to and knowledge about them, and more appreciative of the value of cultural diversity. Cross identifies **cultural pre-competence** as the first positive level on the continuum (the lower levels representing hatred, apathy, and insensitivity). At this level, there is initial recognition of the need for change and understanding in order to relate to others more effectively. **Cultural competence** is a more advanced level on the continuum, with the development of a skill set for dealing with issues related to diversity and cultural differences (Table 7-1). **Cultural proficiency** is on the highest level of the continuum and has been described as an "attitude" rather than a level of knowledge.[12] One does not "achieve" cultural proficiency; it is an ongoing process of learning, reflection, and change.[1]

Cultural Groups and Generalizations

When studying components of culture, it can be helpful to look at how individuals fit into the bigger cultural picture and how people relate to each other. For example, all people need oxygen, nourishment, and water. Under this universal heading are subcategories of attributes that are shared with some but not others. These are such

Table 7-1   Development of Cultural Expertise

Pre-competence	Competence	Proficiency
Acknowledging the presence of similarities and differences between cultures; recognizing weaknesses in one's own skill set	Possessing a set of skills and/or resources to use to function effectively in interactions with those of varying cultural backgrounds	Valuing diversity, continuously striving to gain a better understanding and appreciation of other cultures; making changes in one's approach and attitudes as a result of self-examination and ongoing education

Adapted from Cross et al,[12] as found in *Cross-Cultural Rehabilitation: An International Perspective.*[6]

characteristics as age, gender, ethnicity, and socioeconomic status. Although "members" of each group may share similar characteristics, the individuals remain unique, based on differing biological makeup, personality traits, and life experiences. Trouble arises when individuals are associated with certain groups or cultures without recognizing that:

- Many groupings or "subcultures" may exist within an overall cultural label.[1] For example, immigrants from the same East African country may be of different religious backgrounds.
- A person may identify with a certain group much more strongly than with another. For example, a female's gender may be a much more prominent part of her cultural identity than her ethnicity. For someone else, the opposite may be true.
- A person who is part of a certain group may not practice all the beliefs or have all the characteristics associated with that group. For example, someone may identify herself as Catholic, yet she may use a contraceptive, a violation of church doctrine.[13]

Students will often ask for references regarding the beliefs or practices of a certain cultural group with which they are unfamiliar. Although these lists are available and can be of benefit in preparing students, there is danger in making generalizations about members of a group without taking the individual into consideration.[14] Students should avoid relying on stereotypes and assuming that everyone in the cultural group is as described in a "list" of characteristics. Even without lists, people tend to make assumptions about what they know (or think they know) about cultural groups. For example, most of those reading this textbook would list "college student" as part of their cultural identity. To some, the phrase "college student" brings to mind a person in her late teens, single, no children, living in a dorm during the school year and moving home during the summer, with parents who provide significant financial support. How many of you fit this picture? Probably a few match this description, and others meet parts of it, but many of you probably do not have anything in common with this stereotypical image. For some, "college student" may be the most important component of your current cultural identity, but for others, other cultural components or "roles" (such as that of parent) take precedence.

However, those people who are less familiar with the range in demographics of today's "typical" college student may not be as sensitive to differences. The same is true of any cultural group—less familiarity with individual people of a particular group leads to generalizations about them as all being similar. The result is being less likely to recognize each person's uniqueness and those ways in which that person differs from the stereotypical image that one has developed.

FOR REFLECTION

- For those of you who identified yourself as a college student, think ahead to your graduation ceremony. Your commencement speaker invites all of the new graduates to "stand up, turn around, and thank your parents for their support while you went to school." How would this make you feel? How might your reaction differ depending on how much you associate yourself with the stereotypical "college student" image described earlier?

Biases and Stereotypes

Along with the development of cultural identification, one's upbringing may also be responsible for the development of biases and stereotypes. Most people like to believe they have no biases and view everyone in the most favorable light. However, most people do hold various levels of attitudes or beliefs that interfere with their relationships with other cultural groups.[1,15] People may not be aware that these beliefs (known as **covert bias**) exist or, if they are aware, do not want to acknowledge them because they are embarrassed at having such beliefs. People are usually able to act in ways that do not let their biases influence them. However, in times of stress, they can revert to subconscious behavior, and biases or stereotypes can become more prevalent.[16]

For example, I perform my clinic work in the geriatric setting. I am constantly amazed by the way that many of my clients refuse to "act" old (by my definition of acting old). However, if I am in my car, late for a meeting, and caught behind another car going slower than the speed limit, I have been guilty of saying, "Come on, Grandma, get moving . . ." without even seeing who is driving the car. Do I really rationally think that every slow driver is a senior citizen? No, but at some point my subconscious learned and accepted the stereotype that older people are slower drivers. It may be that this particular belief has a basis in fact, but I am applying it in a way that assumes *all* slow drivers must be old and making it a negative characteristic.

The danger of any type of stereotype is that people make assumptions about what others should be or do based on a "group" into which people have placed them, without taking individuals' characteristics into account.[3] Even positive stereotypes may make someone feel that she is not being judged for who she is as an individual. Suppose I assume that all my female geriatric patients will fit into the "sweet little old lady" stereotype. Am I going to have a harsher view of those patients who are more verbal or emotional if I think that all older women are quiet, calm, and easygoing? I may insult someone or deny someone the opportunity to vent or grieve if I discourage her from acting in a way that does not align with my stereotypical image of how she should act.

Acknowledging the presence of biases and stereotypes is the first step in overcoming their effects.[3] By becoming aware of biases and recognizing that they are generalizations that have been applied to everyone in a group, people are better able to treat each person as an individual with unique attributes.[3]

FOR REFLECTION

- Can you identify any biases or stereotypes you have? What influenced their development? What caused you to recognize them as stereotypes or biases versus facts?

Often the best way to counteract holding a stereotype of a group is by having repeated exposure to individuals in that group. After over 30 years of working with older adults, I find it difficult to hold the stereotype that all older women are sweet little old ladies. Similarly, a person might think that members of a given immigrant population are uneducated or untrained for skilled work because they do not speak English well, only to find when interacting with them individually that many of them speak multiple languages and held prestigious jobs in their native countries. This "learning from exposure" is the theory behind **service learning,** an activity that is becoming common in PT and PTA curricula.[17,18] While performing activities (discussed later in this chapter) with members of various cultural groups, students become more aware of how people within a given culture are individuals, carrying some characteristics of the group but also having their own unique traits. Students then recognize the inappropriateness of universally assigning a given trait to all members of one cultural group.[17-19]

FOR REFLECTION

- Can you think of a stereotype or bias that you held against a certain group or culture that you no longer see as being accurate? What happened to make your opinion change?

Power and Privilege

Cultural interactions are often affected by issues of power and privilege. Having power means that one group (or individual) holds an advantage over another in terms of resources, decision-making, and influence. Groups or individuals with power have the capability to dominate others.[15,20] The dominant cultural group with power has a greater ability to override or ignore the cultural components of the other group. Those without power often feel they have no voice and no ability to demand that their cultural attributes are acknowledged and respected. There are power differentials everywhere. In the classroom, there is a power differential between students and the instructor. In the clinical environment, there is a power differential between patients and providers. The person who is in the position of power has the responsibility to ensure that it is not abused and to empower the other person to use her voice.

Often the cultural group that has power also has privilege. Having **privilege** means that one group is able to assume that its cultural norms and expectations are accepted and supported without having to confirm that to be the case.[14,21] For those without privilege, however, similar actions or behaviors do not have the same level of acceptance, and actions cannot occur without being taken for granted. For example, a heterosexual woman can hold her partner's hand in public without having to worry whether someone will make a derogatory comment. A homosexual woman does not have that privilege. A white male can drive his car through an upper-class neighborhood and not worry he is going to be pulled over by the police. However, an African American male may be much more hesitant to do so, knowing that his odds of being pulled over for no reason are much higher merely based on his race, a situation called "racial profiling."[22] Other types of cultural groups can be said to have privilege if one group has an advantage over another. In any case, it is likely that the disadvantaged group will recognize its lack of privilege more than the privileged group recognizes the benefits it has received.[15]

FOR REFLECTION

FOR REFLECTION

- Think about the different cultural groups to which you belong. Which of these have power and/or privilege and which do not? Can you think of a situation in which you may have received treatment different from that of someone else in that same situation, related to whether or not you had power or privilege?

Health-Care Disparities

The lack of power and privilege can be a factor in the development of **health-care disparities.** A health-care disparity is a situation in which a person has a greater likelihood of developing a certain disease as a result of belonging to a certain ethnic group. For example, those of Native American ethnicity have a higher likelihood of developing diabetes.[14,23,24] Many health-care disparities are related to race, ethnicity, and gender. They may be connected to elements of culture (for example, a traditional diet of a cultural group that is high in fat or sugar) or lifestyle (some cultures may tend to be more physically active than others), but they are more likely to be related to differences in educational level, neighborhood of residence, or other factors with a socioeconomic component.[14,23,25] Those who have lower socioeconomic status generally have poorer access to medical services, health insurance, and even to grocery stores selling healthy meal options (fresh vegetables and meats versus precooked frozen entrees). Unfortunately, certain ethnic groups are more likely to have a lower socioeconomic status, making them more susceptible to being affected by a health-care disparity.[23]

Some health-care disparities may have roots in stereotyping and bias.[14] As an example, one study found that African American men who went to an emergency room complaining of chest pain were more likely than white men to be sent home instead of being admitted for further testing.[26] Health-care providers may be less likely to provide services in certain neighborhoods based on the stereotypes they hold about those neighborhoods.[27] PTs and PTAs must understand that disparities exist and do all that they can in their roles as health-care providers (and as members of society) to promote the development of systems and procedures that help to reduce or eliminate them.[23]

The Culture of Health Care and Physical Therapy

The workplace has a "culture," and health care is no exception. On the first day of each clinical experience, a PTA student typically is shown around the facility, introduced to others, told where to sit, where to put her lunch, and where to find things. This introduction to how things are done at the site is really an introduction to the site's culture, and every site is different. Some routines, also referred to as "norms," may be stated explicitly, such as the work hours. These explicit expectations are called **overt norms.** Other norms, such as the expectation to do paperwork during the lunch hour, may not be stated. These are **covert norms,** expected to be followed even though they have never been expressed. Sometimes covert norms are learned only by asking or by experience.

- Can you think of any overt and covert norms that exist in your classroom?

The U.S. health-care system has a culture of its own, many components of which are not overtly stated to those who are new to it.[1] For example, those who are familiar with it assume they need to:

- Make an appointment when medical care is needed
- Make a copayment at the time of this appointment
- Wait days or weeks to see certain types of medical professionals
- Wait at the appointment for a significant amount of time before being seen (often wearing nothing more than a paper gown)

People new to the U.S. health-care system might not understand or agree with these norms, even after having them made explicit. They can become easily frustrated, especially if these rules are learned through a negative experience. The culture of the U.S. health-care system can therefore become another barrier to diverse populations seeking services and can itself become a factor in health-care discrepancies.[4]

Culturally Appropriate Services

Providing culturally appropriate services means being proactively aware and sensitive to the individual's needs. By acknowledging the patient's culture and how it might affect the rehabilitation program, a clinician is helping to reduce the power differential between the health-care provider and the patient. When a patient believes that her beliefs and values are being acknowledged, she is more likely to participate fully in her rehabilitation.[28] The "golden rule," which is to treat others as one wishes to be treated, has long been considered the standard for interaction. However, it is easy to see that in matters of cultural difference, the assumption that someone wants to be treated the same way as you do is full of potential for conflict and misunderstanding. Another consideration is the use of the "platinum rule," which directs people to "treat others the way *they* would like to be treated."[29] The best way to learn this is to ask questions of the patient (and others, such as family and friends, as appropriate). However, this may not be as simple as it sounds.

Chapter 6 discusses the fact that cultural background can affect how a patient communicates with the health-care provider during times of illness. In addition to the obvious communication barriers created by differences in the languages spoken and understood by the patient and the provider, cultural differences can affect how communication is interpreted, even if the actual words are understood. If a PTA is of a different cultural background from that of the patient, she may interpret the patient's messages differently from the way the patient intends. Some of the components of communication style that have cultural influences include the following:[1]

- A direct instead of an indirect method of communication: In some cultures, getting right to the point in a conversation is efficient. In others, it is offensive to do so, as some relationship-building and "small talk" are expected.
- Gestures, facial expressions, and eye contact can all have different meanings to different groups: Direct eye contact, often considered a sign of respect in traditional Western culture, may be considered inappropriate in others, especially between those of different ages or genders.
- Periods of silence during conversations: Some individuals may need longer processing times than others.
- Titles and last names versus first names: Generational and geographic differences may contribute to patients' expectations with how their names are used and/or how they refer to others.
- Physical touch as part of communication style: Casual touch between "strangers," especially between men and women, may be misinterpreted or considered inappropriate.

Other ways in which culture can affect the patient's participation in the rehabilitation process include the following:

- The patient's belief in the cause and "reason" for the illness: Members of some cultures believe illness is a punishment or a sign from a higher power.
- Who is responsible for decision-making for the patient: In many cultures, others in addition to (or instead of) the patient may be involved.
- The patient's practices of punctuality and timeliness: Arriving "on time" or needing an "appointment" means different things to different people (even within the traditional Western culture).
- How those who are ill should be treated: Members of some cultures believe that people who are ill, disabled, or elderly should be waited on, which can often interfere with the rehabilitation philosophy that patients should do as much for themselves as possible.
- The practice of alternative medical practices: Different cultures may use treatments that may or may not be at odds with Western medical approaches

As with any other skill, developing cultural proficiency and effective cross-cultural communication skills takes practice, and mistakes will be made while learning these skills. However, fear of making or admitting mistakes should not deter clinicians from attempting to improve their skills, as knowledge is gained from any mistake and can be applied to the next situation.[1]

FOR REFLECTION

FOR REFLECTION

- Go back to the scenario at the beginning of the chapter. What were the family's expectations for the delivery of the patient's health-care services? How did those expectations differ from Tyrell's expectations? What could Tyrell do to incorporate the family's wishes into the delivery of the patient's PT interventions?

How to Become More Culturally Competent

Once again, the first step in becoming more culturally competent is to look at yourself and identify your own beliefs, values, and biases.[3] After having done this, do all you can to familiarize yourself with other cultures, especially those with which you will be having frequent contact as patients or coworkers. This can be done by reading, by doing research on the Internet, or by service learning or other volunteer activities. Go to restaurants or shops that are located in ethnically diverse neighborhoods in your community. Learn about some of the issues with which those of different cultural groups are dealing (access to health care, lack of classes to learn English, same-sex partner benefits, human rights violations). Ask questions of your patients or others within another cultural group, and do so in a way that reflects interest, open-mindedness, and the desire to learn.[1] Balance the knowledge of trends within given cultural groups with the characteristics of the individual. These will be learned only by direct interaction with others within those groups.

Service learning was identified previously as a way of helping to recognize the errors of stereotyping. In service-learning activities, students are immersed within a different cultural environment or population, usually one in which they have limited familiarity, to provide some type of needed "service" for that population. However, as opposed to traditional community service activities, they are not there for that reason alone. Students enter the activity with specific learning objectives about themselves, the community, and their role as citizens.[30] By using reflection and reciprocal learning activities with community partners, students often report increased awareness of and respect for the problems faced by individuals who have socioeconomic challenges and limited access to support services. They also report greater awareness of their societal responsibilities as health-care providers and as citizens in minimizing health disparities.[18,30] Finally, research shows that students who participate in service-learning activities strengthen their professional behaviors.[31]

Culturally Competent Interaction Between Colleagues

Up to this point, this chapter has primarily addressed the issue of cultural competency as it affects interaction with patients. Many texts on cultural competence approach the subject with the assumption that the health-care provider is a person of privilege or of the majority. However, the health-care industry is becoming more diverse, and issues of cultural difference between coworkers is becoming more common. Unfortunately, issues of bias continue to be present in the workplace,[4] and the profession of physical therapy is no exception to this.[27]

What should be the response to a colleague (or a patient, for that matter) who makes an overtly culturally insensitive remark? Recognizing that everybody makes mistakes in this area, it might be most appropriate to point out how the comment makes the listener feel, without assigning negative intent. For example, the speaker may not have realized the inappropriateness of the comment and may not be at the same level of cultural competence as the listener. It is important for those who do have power and privilege to speak up when inappropriate comments are made, to help educate others, and to protect the rights of those who have less power and are less comfortable speaking up.

More commonly, issues of bias are more covert. Research has shown that some physical therapy students have been the recipients of covert bias. A study of clinical instructors found that 3.8 percent admitted having lower performance expectations for minority students.[32] Another study had clinicians rate the videotaped performance of a "student" presenting a report to a physician. One of four different tapes was randomly viewed by each participant. Each tape used the same script, but the race and/or ethnicity of the student was different in each tape (black, white, Asian, and Hispanic). The results of the study found that the black student consistently received lower scores than the other students regarding the clarity of her presentation, her ability to hold the listener's interest, and the thoroughness and organization of her report, despite having given the same report as the others. The white student received more negative comments about the content of her report, yet still received a higher overall rating than the black student. The researchers noted that the black student had a significant accent compared with the other speakers; they recognized that this could have affected the viewers' interpretation of her presentation compared with that of the other students.[33]

Who has the power or privilege if the PTA is a person of a minority background and the patient is a person of the majority? The PTA still has the responsibility as the person of power in the patient/provider relationship to ensure that differences of culture do not interfere with patient performance and progress. For example, if a PTA has an accent, she must ensure that the patient feels empowered to ask her to repeat directions if the patient is not able to understand her because of the PTA's accent. If issues of culture appear to be interfering with the delivery of interventions, regardless of who is the member of the majority culture, the PTA should look to her supervising PT for assistance in resolving the issues.

FOR REFLECTION

- How would you respond to a fellow student or coworker who says, "I am 'color blind.' I treat everyone the same. After all, we are all alike on the inside." Do you agree that this is the way we should treat others?

Spirituality

Spirituality is another extremely personal topic and a component of culture that many people are uncomfortable discussing with others. It is one example of a cultural component that can be fluid throughout life. Religious and spiritual beliefs can often come to the forefront during times of illness, especially if the illness is particularly challenging or life-threatening.[3,34,35] In physical therapy, the focus has tended to be on the physical side of functioning, yet studies show that patients are able to deal with physical limitations better if they are at ease spiritually.[35,36] Many physical therapy educational programs do not contain significant classroom content on the topic of spirituality,[37] and although clinicians appear to recognize its influence on healing, many do not feel comfortable with or prepared for having conversations about spirituality with their patients.[36]

Most experts differentiate between religion and spirituality, although the two can certainly overlap. Religion is more often related to a belief in a specific higher power and includes structured rules or external rituals that people practice as part of their faith beliefs. Spirituality is less concrete and is more an internal process used to develop a sense of wellness and to help find meaning and purpose in life.[34,38] Someone can have a strong sense of spirituality with or without practicing the beliefs of an organized religion.[34] As physical therapy focuses more and more on providing services promoting wellness, clinicians in this area of practice may also be challenged to address spirituality as a component of wellness.[38]

As part of the response to illness or injury, patients may express a loss of faith or anger at a higher power for "giving" them an illness. They may question why that higher power is "keeping them alive" if their self-perceived quality of life is poor. The PTA should attempt to develop proficiency in addressing these types of comments because it reinforces that she is concerned for the patient as a whole, not just the patient's impairments or functional limitations.[3,35] The process for improving skills in this area is similar to that of developing cultural competency. The first step is to look at your own beliefs and values in the area of spirituality. This will help you to be more comfortable in acknowledging issues of spirituality and more sensitive to differences you might have with others' beliefs. The next step is to familiarize yourself with religious and spiritual practices that differ from your own. Ask questions of the patient, the family, or others with expertise in spirituality. Familiarity in the subject matter will also help you to be more sensitive to the patient's own beliefs and outward expressions of faith.[38]

The PTA should not minimize the patient's feelings or offer false hope in times of terminal illness. However, many times the patient may just need acknowledgment of her emotions, which often can be provided by active listening skills (see Chapter 6).[35] Some patients will ask about a provider's beliefs. The provider should be prepared for this, deciding ahead of time whether she is able and willing to discuss them. Of course, this should be done only if the patient initiates the conversation and only if the provider is comfortable doing so.[34] If not, or if she does not feel she can address the patient's concerns, the PTA should discuss the issue with the supervising PT. It may be more appropriate to refer the patient to a facility chaplain or other member of the clergy, to social services, or to another type of psychosocial counseling.[34]

FOR REFLECTION

- If a patient asked you to pray with her, would you be comfortable doing so? Why or why not?

S U M M A R Y

The United States is becoming increasingly more culturally diverse, and cultural competence is an increasingly important skill set required for effective interaction with patients, families, coworkers, and classmates. Recognizing our own beliefs, values, and biases is a necessary step in developing competence in dealing with issues of culture and spirituality. In learning about other cultures, we must remember to consider the individual within the context of generalizations related to cultural groups. Cultural differences related to socioeconomics are a key component in the ongoing problem of health disparities in the United States, but improvements in culturally competent care will play a role in helping to eliminate disparities. Each of us must strive to achieve cultural proficiency, an ongoing state in which valuing and supporting a variety of cultures becomes second nature.

R E F E R E N C E S

1. Black JD, Purnell LD. Cultural competence for the physical therapy professional. *J Phys Ther Educ*. 2002;16(1):3-10.
2. Padilla R, Brown K. Culture and patient education: challenges and opportunities. *J Phys Ther Educ*. 1999;13(3):23-30.
3. Lattanzi JB, Purnell LD. *Developing Cultural Competence in Physical Therapy Practice.* Philadelphia, PA: FA Davis; 2006:417.
4. Purnell LD, Paulanka BJ. *Transcultural Health Care: A Culturally Competent Approach.* 4th ed. Philadelphia, PA: FA Davis; 2013:480.
5. US Census Bureau. Overview of race and hispanic origin: 2010. 2010 Census Briefs Web site. http://www.census.gov/prod/cen2010/briefs/c2010br-02.pdf. Updated 2011. Accessed August 17, 2015.
6. Leavitt R, ed. *Cross-Cultural Rehabilitation: An International Perspective.* Philadelphia, PA: WB Saunders; 1999.
7. Commission on Accreditation in Physical Therapy Education. 2012-2013 fact sheet: physical therapist assistant programs. http://www.capteonline.org/uploadedFiles/CAPTEorg/About_CAPTE/Resources/Aggregate_Program_Data/AggregateProgramData_PTAPrograms.pdf. Updated 2013. Accessed August 10, 2015.
8. Commission on Accreditation in Physical Therapy Education. 2014-15 physical therapist education programs fact sheets. http://www.capteonline.org/uploadedFiles/CAPTEorg/About_CAPTE/Resources/Aggregate_Program_Data/AggregateProgramData_PTPrograms.pdf. Updated 2015. Accessed August 17, 2015.
9. Wojciechowski M. Juggling the unique aspects of PTA education. *PT in Motion*. 2013;5(3).
10. American Physical Therapy Association. Operational plan on cultural competence. http://www.apta.org/uploadedFiles/APTAorg/About_Us/Policies/APTA_Adopted_Plans/OperationalPlanCulturalCompetence.pdf. Updated 2012. Accessed August 17, 2015.

11. American Physical Therapy Association. Minority scholarship award. http://www.apta.org/HonorsandAwards/Scholarships/MinorityScholarship/. Updated 2015. Accessed August 17, 2015.
12. Cross TL, Bazron BJ, Dennis KW, Isaacs MR. *Towards a Culturally Competent System of Health Care.* Vol 1. Washington, DC: Georgtown University Press; 1989.
13. Pope Paul VI. Encyclical letter: Humanae vitae. 1968.
14. Leavitt RL, Leavitt RL. Developing cultural competence in a multicultural world part I. *PT Magazine.* 2002;10(12):36.
15. Tatum BD. *Why Are All the Black Kids Sitting Together in the Cafeteria? And Other Conversations About Race.* New York, NY: Basic Books; 1999:270.
16. Burgess DJ, Fu SS, van Ryn M. Why do providers contribute to disparities and what can be done about it? *J Gen Intern Med.* 2004;19(11):1154-1159.
17. Village D, Clouten N, Millar AL, et al. Comparison of the use of service learning, volunteer and pro bono activities in physical therapy curricula. *J Phys Ther Educ.* 2004;1(22):28.
18. Brosky JA, Deprey SM, Hopp JF, Maher EJ. Physical therapist student and community partner perspectives and attitudes regarding service-learning experiences. *J Phys Ther Educ.* 2006;20(3):41-54.
19. Beling J. Impact of service learning on physical therapist students' knowledge of and attitudes toward older adults and on their critical thinking ability. *J Phys Ther Educ.* 2004;18(1):13-21.
20. Tatum BD. *Can We Talk About Race? And Other Conversations in an Era of School Resegregation.* Boston, MA: Beacon Press; 2007:147.
21. McIntosh P. White privilege: unpacking the invisible knapsack. *Independent Sch.* 1990;49(2):31.
22. American Civil Liberties Union. Racial profiling: definition. https://www.aclu.org/racial-profiling-definition. Updated 2015. Accessed August 17, 2015.
23. Kosoko-Lasaki S, Cook CT, O'Brian RL. *Cultural Proficiency in Addressing Health Disparities.* Sudbury, MA: Jones & Bartlett; 2009:433.
24. Cochran TM, Curtis CT, eds. *Rehabilitation and American Indian Elders.* Alexandria, VA: American Physical Therapy Association; 2003; No. 3.
25. Leavitt RL, Leavitt RL. Developing cultural competence in a multicultural world part II. *PT Magazine.* 2003;11(1):56.
26. Pezzin LE, Pezzin LE, Keyl PM, Green GB. Disparities in the emergency department evaluation of chest pain patients. *Acad Emerg Med.* 2007;14(2):149-156.
27. Royeen M, Crabtree J. *Culture in Rehabilitation: From Competency to Proficiency.* Upper Saddle River, NJ: Pearson Prentice Hall; 2006:386.
28. Ekelman B, Bello-Haas VD, Bazyk J, Bazyk S. Developing cultural competence in occupational therapy and physical therapy education: a field immersion approach. *J Allied Health.* 2003;32(2):131-137.
29. Alessandra T. The platinum rule. http://www.alessandra.com/abouttony/aboutpr.asp. Updated 2015. Accessed August 17, 2015.
30. Reynolds PJ. Commentary and introduction: service learning and community-engaged scholarship. *J Phys Ther Educ.* 2006;20(3):3-7.

31. Wise HH, Yuen HK. Effect of community-based service learning on professionalism in student physical therapists. *J Phys Ther Educ*. 2013;27(2):58-64.
32. Clouten N, Homma M, Shimada R. Clinical education and cultural diversity in physical therapy: clinical performance of minority student physical therapists and the expectations of clinical instructors. *Physiother Theory Pract*. 2006;22(1): 1-15.
33. Haskins AR, Rose-St. Prix C, Elbaum L. Covert bias in evaluation of physical therapist students' clinical performance. *Phys Ther*. 1997;77(2):155-163.
34. Coyne C. Addressing spirituality issues in patient interventions. *PT Magazine*. 2005;13(7):38-44.
35. Johansson C. Rising with the fall: addressing quality of life in physical frailty. *Top Geriatr Rehabil*. 2003;19(4):239-248.
36. Oakley ET, Katz G, Sauer K, Dent B, Millar AL. Physical therapists' perception of spirituality and patient care: beliefs, practices, and perceived barriers. *J Phys Ther Educ*. 2010;24(2):45-52.
37. Pitts J. Spirituality in the physical therapy curriculum: effects on the older adult. *Top Geriatr Rehabil*. 2008;24(4):281-294.
38. Sargeant DM. Teaching spirituality in the physical therapy classroom and clinic. *J Phys Ther Educ*. 2009;23(1):29-35.

Name _____

REVIEW

1. Explain the difference between primary and secondary cultural characteristics.

_____

_____

_____

_____

_____

2. List and describe three ways in which your preferred methods of communication might differ from those of someone else in another cultural group:

a. _____

_____

b. _____

_____

c. _____

_____

Application

1. Review the concept of privilege and the examples of it as described in this chapter. Give one additional example of how a different cultural characteristic could contribute to someone having/not having privilege.

_____

_____

_____

_____

(questions continue on page 140)

2. Identify one health disparity involving members of an ethnic group you may work with during your various clinical experiences. List three to four factors that might be contributing to the perpetuation of the disparity.

_____

_____

_____

_____

3. You are working with an older woman in a skilled nursing facility. One day, when you arrive at her room, she starts to cry and says, "This isn't working. I'm not going to get any better. Why won't God just let me die?" How would you respond to this patient?

_____

_____

_____

_____

8

Introduction to Documentation for the Physical Therapist Assistant

CHAPTER OBJECTIVES

After reading the chapter, the reader will be able to:

- Explain the various purposes for which documentation is used.
- List the basic principles of proper physical therapy documentation.
- Describe the content included in each section of the SOAP (subjective, objective, assessment, and plan) note.
- Discuss commonly seen documentation formats.
- Give examples of components of documentation that can and cannot be performed by the physical therapist assistant (PTA), according to American Physical Therapy Association (APTA) and/or third-party payer guidelines.
- Identify APTA resources for improving documentation skills.
- Discuss common problems in documentation.
- Recite the top 10 reasons for payment denials related to documentation as identified by the APTA.

KEY TERMS AND CONCEPTS

- Progress note
- SOAP
- Subjective
- Objective
- Assessment
- Goals/outcomes
- Plan

- Source-oriented format
- Problem-oriented format
- Narrative note
- Flow sheet
- Electronic health record (EHR)
- "Defensible Documentation for Patient/Client Management"

S*henice, an experienced PTA, is attending a patient care conference at the skilled nursing facility in which she works part-time. She is asked to give an update on the patient's ability to go up and down stairs, as the patient will need to*

(vignette continues on page 142)

perform this independently upon discharge to his home. Shenice remembers that she had practiced the stairs with the patient a couple of days ago, but she does not recall how well the patient did. As she looks back on her charting, she is dismayed to see that her notes from that day merely say, "Pt. ↑↓ stairs 2." The patient insists that he is able to go up and down stairs independently, and Shenice is asked to verify this. Shenice quickly reviews the notes of the other clinicians who worked with the patient on the days she was not working, but she sees no documentation about stairs.

QUESTIONS TO CONSIDER

How could Shenice's documentation have been more complete regarding the patient's performance on the stairs? What information is missing? Should Shenice assume that no one else has practiced going up and down stairs with this patient? If the patient is discharged and later falls while on the stairs at home, would this level of documentation support any claim that the patient was discharged before he could safely be independent?

For many clinicians, completing the paperwork involved with the provision of physical therapy services is the least favorite part of their day. Most people in this career decided to pursue it in part because of a preference for being active instead of doing work at a desk. However, documentation is a necessity in health care, and being able to accurately document what happens in a given intervention session is as important a skill for the PTA to develop as those techniques performed directly with the patient. Like those other skills, it requires practice and feedback in order to improve on it. However, the fast pace of today's clinical environment may contribute to cutting corners on documentation and being less thorough than would be appropriate. The advent of electronic documentation, although a potential time saver, also may lend itself to using certain phrases routinely without enough detail to support the need for skilled services. If documentation is not performed in a clear, complete manner that reflects the level of skill required by the person providing the intervention, it can affect payment for the services delivered. Substandard documentation could be used against a clinician in a legal case seeking to show inappropriate care. In a worst-case scenario, it could even be used to substantiate a criminal complaint of fraud!

This chapter is intended to serve as a basic overview of the concepts relating to why and how physical therapists (PTs) and PTAs perform documentation, not to develop expertise in creating appropriate documentation. As stated, that skill takes much practice and is an ongoing process. Many textbooks focus solely on developing documentation skills, and this chapter is not meant to replace those. Rather, it reviews the purposes for which documentation is used and discusses the basic principles of how to document correctly when writing progress notes (daily or weekly documentation of the patient's current status) using one of the most basic documentation styles, the SOAP note format. This chapter also discusses the ways in which the PTA's role in performing documentation may differ from that of the PT, based on requirements of state practice acts, the APTA, and third-party payers. Finally, the chapter briefly reviews other documentation formats, discusses common problems in documentation, and introduces the reader to the APTA's "Defensible Documentation for Patient/Client Management," an online resource for improving documentation skills.

Purposes of Documentation

An old adage in health care states, "If it isn't documented, it didn't happen." The primary purpose of documentation is to serve as a record of everything that occurred in a given day's intervention session. However, documentation serves many other purposes as well. Other reasons for performing documentation include the following:

- Supporting the need for skilled therapy services
- Substantiating the charges that were billed for that particular day's intervention
- Providing a record of different interventions that were used with a patient (and the outcomes associated with them) throughout a complete episode of care
- Providing a record of improvement or lack of improvement related to the patient's impairments, functional limitations, and disabilities
- Giving a rationale to explain why a patient may not be improving as quickly as expected
- Serving as a tool to be used in the performance of retroactive research, peer review, and quality outcomes measurement to support evidence-based practice and the services provided
- Providing a legal record of the episode of care

Documentation Standards and Principles

Documentation can be performed in various formats and styles. It can be handwritten or completed electronically, using a free-flowing narrative style or using a checklist-type flow sheet designed for a particular patient diagnosis. But because it is a legal record, certain standards and principles should be followed, no matter what format is used, to maintain its quality and validity.

Style

As opposed to traditional writing, medical documentation is usually not as wordy. Sentence structure is somewhat abbreviated, and less descriptive wording is used. It is not unusual to see sentences in which the subject is implied, not stated, or sentences that would be considered run-ons or fragments if used in other writing formats. For example, a phrase summarizing how a patient described his previous night's sleep might read, "Reports taking Ibuprofen (400 mg) prior to bed, woke up × 1 due to pain, able to get back to sleep without additional medication during night." In medical documentation, this concise style of writing is considered acceptable, even though it may not be grammatically correct, because it allows the writer to save time and get to the point of the note quickly.

At the same time, documentation needs to be clear and complete. If a note is written that is too brief or too concise, key points may be left out or may not be interpreted accurately. A note that is too short or not descriptive enough may fail to support the need for the skilled services being provided. In electronic documentation, frequent use of key phrases in documentation templates often result in "note cloning," in which patient notes all appear very similar.[1] Students are generally encouraged to write more rather than less when they are learning the art of documentation to help them develop good habits of inclusion. With experience, it becomes easier to become more concise without sacrificing quality.

FOR REFLECTION

- A progress note includes the sentence "Pt. performed hip exercises." What other information needs to be included about the hip exercises to make the note more complete?

Abbreviations

Many commonly used medical abbreviations are derived from Latin words and phrases. For example, the abbreviation BID comes from the Latin phrase *bis in die*, which means "twice daily."[2] Therefore, if someone is receiving physical therapy two times per day, they are said to be seen BID. Other abbreviations come from a shortening of the word in English, such as "pt." for "patient," or the initials of a term or phrase, such as "PT" for "physical therapy." In some cases, symbols such as "↑" or "↓" might be used to substitute for the words "up" and "down" or "increased" and "decreased."

The last two examples show some of the problems that can occur with the use of abbreviations. Many abbreviations can represent more than one term. For example, in addition to "patient" and "physical therapy," "PT" could also be used to refer to a type of blood test (prothrombin time), an amount of blood transfused (pint), or the type of metal used in a prosthetic joint (platinum, using its abbreviation from the periodic table).[1] Often, the context in which the abbreviation is used will make it clear what it represents, but not always. More than once in this author's experience, a supposed order from a physician for physical therapy has turned out to be an order for a prothrombin time test!

Most facilities will have a list of approved abbreviations that can be used within the documentation written by their employees. However, documentation frequently is shared beyond the facility with others who will not have access to that abbreviation list. If there is any doubt about whether those who subsequently read the documentation will know or understand the abbreviation, it should not be used.

FOR REFLECTION
FOR REFLECTION

■ How could you rewrite the following sentences so that they are more concise, while still containing all pertinent information? Are there any abbreviations that would be appropriate to use in rewriting these sentences? If possible, compare your rewritten note with one that someone else has rewritten.

The patient ambulated across the clinic for a distance of 100 feet, using a standard walker. He used a slow pace and required minimal assistance to pick up the walker, move it forward, and position it so that all four walker legs touched down at the same time. The patient also needed to be reminded to stand up straight and to take longer steps. While the patient was ambulating, he complained of pain in his right and left hips.

Errors

Despite our best efforts, there will be times when a mistake is made while writing a patient note. When this occurs, it should be corrected in a manner consistent with how other legal documents are corrected. In handwritten documentation, errors should never be erased, scribbled out, or covered with white eraser fluid. The writer should draw a single line through the incorrect word and write the word "error" above or next to the mistake, along with the writer's initials and the date. By correcting an error in this manner, the mistake can still be read and the reader can be assured that the legal record has not been inappropriately altered. The process differs slightly in electronic documentation formats, as notes can usually be corrected while they are in the process of being written. Once officially entered, however, they may not be able to be changed. In either format, if additional information needs to be included later, or an error is noted at a later time after the writer has completed the note, some type of addendum at the bottom of the note or on a separate page should be used to add to or correct the original information.

Dates

All documentation should be dated. Depending on the documentation format, the date may appear at the start of the note or at the bottom alongside the clinician's signature. If a note is being written at a date later than when the intervention was delivered (e.g., in a situation when the clinician has forgotten to write a note about an intervention session), the phrase "late entry" is often used to denote this.

Signatures

All documentation must be signed by the author, along with the abbreviation representing his regulatory title (i.e., Holly Clynch, PT), not the clinician's earned physical therapy degree (Holly Clynch, DPT). Depending on state law, notes written by a PTA may need to be cosigned by a PT. When students perform documentation, it should always be cosigned by the supervising clinician. The letter *S*, for student, is commonly added ("SPTA" or "SPT") to indicate student status.

Black Ink

Patient notes are legal documents, so it is expected that handwritten documentation will be done in black ink. However, as the quality of photocopies continues to improve, it has become more common to see blue ink required for signatures on legal documents to better differentiate between copies and originals. This is not common practice in physical therapy at this time; use of black ink for handwritten documentation continues to be the norm. Pencil should never be used on documentation because of the potential that it could be changed by erasure.

Third Person

References to self should be used infrequently because the focus of the documentation should be on the patient and not on the clinician. However, sometimes the clinician may need to refer to himself when writing a note. This should always be done in third-person format, using "this PTA" or "this clinician" rather than using "I" or "me."

Documentation Content

Depending on the setting and third-party payer requirements, documentation of patient interventions, referred to as **progress notes,** can be written on a daily basis, a weekly basis, or within other time frames as decided on by the facility. Regardless of the format used (examples are discussed in following sections in this chapter) or how often the note is required, the standard content contained within a given progress note is generally the same. Progress notes should all contain the following:

- Information reported to the clinician, observed by the clinician, or performed by/ with the patient during the intervention session
- The clinician's reflection/judgment concerning how the patient's present status relates to the anticipated progress and expected outcomes of the therapy interventions
- Suggestions about what needs to occur (either by the patient or the provider) to promote further progress and achievement of patient outcomes

The acronym **SOAP** is used to refer to the traditional style of organizing this information. SOAP stands for **s**ubjective, **o**bjective, **a**ssessment, and **p**lan. Each of these sections differs from the others because of the type of information found within it.

Subjective

In the **subjective** section, the writer documents information relevant to the patient's episode of care told to the writer by other people. These sources may include the patient, the patient's family, other members of the patient's health-care team, or anyone else connected with the patient. It may or may not be accurate, hence the use of the term "subjective." This section might include such things as the patient's opinion of how he is progressing, his statements regarding where and how much pain he is having, reports from others on what they have observed the patient doing when not in physical therapy, or records of conversations the writer may have had with other health-care professionals regarding the patient's diagnosis or discharge plans. If using a direct quote from someone, the information should be bracketed by quotation marks. It is more common, however, for the writer to paraphrase what the other person said, in which case quotation marks are not needed. In either case, the source of the information should be made clear, usually by indication of the person's role (i.e., "patient's spouse," "evening shift nursing staff"), although formally naming the source may at times be appropriate or necessary.

Objective

The **objective** section in the progress note is more or less the step-by-step report of what occurred during a given intervention session (or in those intervention sessions delivered since the last note was written, in the case of a weekly review note). It should include a description of the interventions delivered and the patient's performance level during the delivery of those interventions. The goal of this section is to paint a clear, accurate picture of what occurred in that intervention session and the patient's current level of performance related to his functional abilities. Therefore, when writing this section, it is important to keep the information factual and reproducible. Anything included in this section should be information that another clinician could replicate or observe when working with this patient at the next visit. The results of any tests or measurements taken should also be included in this section, although the relevance of the results should be addressed later in the note.

As part of the description of the patient's status, the writer should address the type of education given and the amount of assistance provided to the patient during his performance of a given task or exercise. This is an area in which some clinicians do not provide enough detail. The PTA must remember that the person reading the note may not be familiar with physical therapy techniques or know how PTs/PTAs help patients to improve their skills. Specific information should be included to reflect the unique observation and physical or education techniques (the "skilled services," in third-party payer jargon) used by the PT or PTA throughout the patient's intervention session. For example, when working with a patient on his gait skills, the PTA should specify any verbal or physical assistance given (i.e., required verbal cues to increase step length in 50% of steps taken, needed moderate assistance to advance wheeled walker) and objectively describe anything that interfered with the patient's ability to perform the task with less assistance (demonstrated loss of balance 3 during gait; required assistance to regain balance × 2).

FOR REFLECTION
FOR REFLECTION

- As noted, information regarding what the patient tells you about his level of pain should be documented in the subjective section. However, if this information is obtained using a numerical pain scale rating ("Please rate your pain on a scale of 0–10, with 0 being no pain and 10 being the worst pain imaginable . . ."), why wouldn't it be placed in the objective section?

Assessment

The **assessment** section is probably the most important section, and it is also the most challenging for many students (and clinicians) to write effectively. In this section, the writer needs to interpret the relevance of the information already presented in the previous sections of the note. It is often helpful to think of this section as answering these questions: So what? Why is this information important? Why does this patient need the services of physical therapy? The writer needs to demonstrate connections between the information presented in the subjective and objective sections and then use those connections to make skilled judgments regarding the effectiveness of the interventions delivered, the patient's response to the interventions, and the need for continued skilled services. Why is the assessment section so important? Insurers who review progress notes need to be able to identify the reason for physical therapy intervention. If it is not clear that the skilled services of the PT/PTA were in fact needed, or if the patient does not appear to be making progress, payment for the services delivered may be denied. This is the section in which this need should be clearly stated.

In the assessment section of a note, the PTA should reflect upon the patient's progress toward the anticipated goals and expected outcomes for each patient, as established by the PT in the patient's plan of care. The *Guide to Physical Therapist Practice* defines a **goal** as "the intended impact on functioning (body functions and structures, activities, participation) as a result of implementing the plan of care." Goals also should be "measurable, functionally driven, and time limited," with anticipated results described in both long-term and short-term time frames.[3] **Outcomes,** the actual results that are achieved as a result of the episode of care, are often broader and more global in nature.[3] If the patient is progressing and has met interim goals, the assessment section of the PTA's note should state this. If the patient has not met his goals, the writer should include his opinion (based on his skill as a PTA and the information already presented in the subjective and objective sections) as to why the goals have not been met.

In developing the plan of care, the PT is clearly responsible for determining the overall goals and outcomes expected by the end of the entire episode of care. The PT is also responsible for modifying any of these goals if they become inappropriate or need to be advanced further. However, it is common for more achievable, interim short-term goals to be set as "stepping stones" that indicate progression toward the overall long-term goals and outcomes. Although PTAs should not be developing the overall goals and outcomes, it is appropriate for a PTA, as part of his documentation of the results of a given patient encounter, to identify objectives and outcomes to be achieved in the next intervention session that will allow the patient to demonstrate progress toward the larger goals.[4]

Some PTs and PTAs (often in response to facility or third-party documentation policies) will occasionally have to defend that a PTA is qualified and/or allowed to write the assessment section of a progress note. Part of the controversy is related to the varying usage and definitions of the word "assessment." However, the APTA's document "Minimum Required Skills of Physical Therapist Assistant Graduates at Entry-Level" lists "Assessment of Patient Response" as an expectation during delivery of interventions.[5] In addition, the *Normative Model of Physical Therapist Assistant Education* clearly states that the PTA should be expected to "provide information in the assessment section based on information gathered from subjective and objective data that will be useful to the physical therapist in evaluating the patient's/client's progress."[6]

Plan

The **plan** section describes what will happen in the future. This may include a description of what might be emphasized in upcoming intervention sessions, equipment that needs to be ordered, or interaction that needs to occur with other health-care professionals. For the PTA, this section would also indicate a need for further consultation with the supervising PT, if appropriate. Often the goals may be reiterated in this section as a way of summarizing the plan. However, as stated, the patient's progress toward those goals should have already been addressed in the assessment section.

FOR REFLECTION

- Go back to the scenario at the beginning of this chapter and review Shenice's documentation. How could she have improved what was written? What additional information could have been included to paint a more accurate picture of the patient's functional ability on the stairs?

Documentation Formats and Organizational Styles

Progress notes may be formatted or organized in various ways. Most formats still use the SOAP note characteristics but present the content in a different manner. A few of these formats are described in the following sections. However, this is *not* intended to be a comprehensive discussion.

Source-Oriented and Problem-Oriented Formats

The **source-oriented** and **problem-oriented formats** represent different ways that notes might be organized within a given facility. In the source-oriented format, the various departments within a health-care facility write their own notes for a patient, and these notes are filed within a patient's chart based on which discipline, or source, wrote the note. For example, physical therapy would have its own section (or would be included within the rehabilitation section of a patient's chart), nursing would have a different section, nutrition another, and so on. Notes in each of these sections might address similar issues, based on the perspective of that discipline. The problem-oriented format differs in that notes written about the patient are categorized based on the patient's diagnosis, goals, or problems, and different disciplines all address each problem within that problem's specific section. For example, multiple departments (nursing, occupational therapy, speech-language pathology, nutrition, etc.) might all be addressing concerns related to a patient's problem of being unable to feed himself independently following a cerebrovascular accident. Sometimes a combination of these formats can be seen. In some facilities, rehabilitation may have its own section within a patient chart, but at times may make entries in an interdisciplinary section in which various departments contribute documentation.

Narrative Notes

In a **narrative note,** the information is usually presented in a more traditional writing format. Although the information may still be laid out following a SOAP-format style, the sections are generally not labeled as such. This format may be used more when describing a specific incident that requires documentation, such as a patient fall or a conversation with a family member, and may include more complete sentences than would the traditional progress note.

Flow Sheets

The **flow sheet** is designed to facilitate quick documentation and requires a minimum of sentence-style writing. It also allows the reader to easily review a number of intervention sessions, as the flow sheet is frequently organized so that the notes for multiple visits are included on one page in a column-style format. Traditionally, the flow sheet includes boxes that can be checked off to indicate status or blanks to be filled in. These boxes or lines are often of limited size, which means that the writer must be extremely concise and write very small. A valid concern about the use of flow sheets is that the limited space within boxes might inhibit the writer from being as precise or as detailed as he might need to be to fully describe how the physical therapy service was delivered or to justify the need for skilled services. Some flow sheets have lines on the back where additional information can be documented in a narrative style, if needed, to alleviate this concern.

Electronic Health Records

It is becoming much more common for facilities to use an **electronic health record (EHR)** (currently the most accepted title, considered to be more inclusive than the electronic medical record, or EMR).[7] The goal of the EHR is to allow for health-related information to be accessible across multiple health-care organizations.[8] Students are likely to have exposure to some type of EHR format at most of their clinical experiences. In response to a 2004 executive order by President Bush supporting "widespread adoption" of EHRs by 2014, the APTA passed a 2006 position that encouraged the use of EHRs in all practice settings.[9] In addition, the American Recovery and Reinvestment Act of 2009 included financial incentives, through Medicare and Medicaid, to health-care providers and facilities who could demonstrate "meaningful use" of EHRs for their patients.[10] At the time of this writing, although many facilities have fully completed the transition to electronic documentation (especially in larger health-care organizations), some are still using paper documentation or a combination of both.

The types of EHR software vary among facilities, and a review of these systems is beyond the scope of this text. Some of the advantages of converting to an EHR include the following:[7,8,11]

- Ease in storing and accessing patient information
- Integrated data collection that contributes to more appropriate clinical decisions
- Improved legibility of entries, leading to more accurate care and improved patient safety, therefore promoting better patient outcomes
- Improved access to current clinical evidence and patient care guidelines
- Improved consistency of billing related to documentation (some systems have automatic reminders or connections between what is documented and what is charged to the patient for a given intervention).

The drawbacks include varying challenges in navigating a given system, the number of hours required to train staff, variations in employee comfort with using computerized systems, the number of computers needed, and the need for a qualified technical support staff.[8] Ironically, improved legibility of documentation in the EMR has actually led to an increase in chart auditing and denial of claims; in the past, records that were less legible were more likely to have been accepted as appropriate.[1] In addition, the previously mentioned use of templates resulting in nonpatient-specific documentation also can result in an increase in claim denials.[1]

In theory, in the future a patient could have all of his medical history and documentation of his current medical care stored electronically in a format that would allow him to transport it to any facility in which he receives care, ensuring that all of his medical providers have full access to any needed information. However, issues related to how information is shared or kept confidential (and who, beyond the patient, has the right and responsibility to store this information), along with poor compatibility between current EMR systems and the still-unknown financial return on investment for a facility implementing an EHR, have interfered with this vision becoming a reality.[5]

Increasingly, clinicians are expected to complete their documentation at the same time that they deliver patient services, a concept known as point-of-care documentation. Electronic documentation systems, especially via devices such as tablets or laptops, have facilitated the ease of doing this.[8] Again, however, structured checklists or drop-down templates, although saving time, can contribute to a lack of specificity in a given patient's note or cause excessive repetition when comparing records of multiple patients.[1]

Interdisciplinary Assessment Tools

A PTA may be asked to record information related to a patient's performance and frequency of participation in physical therapy, which is then used to measure overall functional status and possibly to determine the amount of payment that a facility will receive for provided services. Assessment tools that are used for such measurements include the Minimum Data Set (MDS), which is used in skilled nursing facilities, and the Functional Independence Measure (FIM), frequently used in inpatient rehabilitation. In addition, a PTA may participate in administering standardized screening tests (e.g., the Berg Balance Scale) in which a patient's level of ability in performing certain tasks is given an objective numerical rating, but the interpretation of the total score's meaning (in terms of level of risk or overall functional status) is still considered to be the responsibility of the PT as a component of reexamination.[12]

Roles of the PT and PTA in Documentation

Once again, specific state practice acts may dictate documentation responsibilities or may contain a list of documentation duties that cannot be delegated to the PTA. The APTA also has guidelines and position statements that describe these differences in responsibilities.[3,13] In addition, third-party payer regulations may also make reference to who is allowed to perform certain components of physical therapy documentation. As reiterated in previous chapters, these regulatory bodies may not always be consistent in what they allow or disallow. However, in general terms, the types of documentation that should be completed only by the PT follow in the next sections.

Initial Examinations and Evaluations

Because only the PT can perform these components of patient/client management, the PT must also be the person completing the corresponding documentation. Only documentation of subsequent intervention sessions or a review of a series of intervention sessions, such as in a weekly progress note, may be completed by the PTA.

Development and Modifications of the Initial Plan of Care

Determining the patient's physical therapy diagnosis and prognosis and developing the patient's plan of care are also the sole responsibility of the PT. Any changes to the initial plan of care must be done by the PT. However, PTAs should be able to recognize the need for possible modification to an existing plan of care. If a PTA working with a patient has questions related to the established plan of care, he should discuss those concerns with the supervising PT to best serve the needs of the patient.

Review of Episode of Care at Discharge

The PT is responsible for summarizing the patient's episode of care from beginning to end, documenting the effectiveness of the interventions delivered and the patient's overall progress related to the goals and outcomes set by the PT. But what happens if a patient is unexpectedly discharged, and the PTA was the last person to have worked with that patient? This is a frequent occurrence in physical therapy and has been used by some clinicians to justify having PTAs write discharge documentation. However, the most appropriate course of action in this situation is to have the PTA write a progress note (sometimes referred to as a "discharge note") in which the patient's status on that last day is thoroughly documented without review of the entire episode of care. The review and assessment of the patient's progression throughout the episode of care is then subsequently completed by the PT, using the information provided in the discharge note to indicate the patient's status when last seen.

Components of Third-Party Payer Documentation

Examples of third-party payer documentation requirements can be found in the Medicare system. Medicare has specific forms that are often required to be completed to receive payment for services. Most of these forms include some type of evaluation or reevaluation component, the reason they should be completed only by the PT. Another example of Medicare documentation requirements currently affecting the PTA is the Medicare Part B requirement that the PT (and not the PTA) write a "Progress Report" on the day of the patient's 10th visit and every 10 visits thereafter.[14]

Documentation Authority for Physical Therapy Services (HOD P05-07-09-03)

Physical therapy examination, evaluation, diagnosis, prognosis, and plan of care (including interventions) shall be documented, dated, and authenticated by the physical therapist who performs the service. Interventions provided by the physical therapist or selected interventions provided by the physical therapist assistant under the direction and supervision of the physical therapist are documented, dated, and authenticated by the physical therapist or, when permissible by law, the physical therapist assistant. Other notations or flow charts are considered a component of the documented record but do not meet the requirements of documentation in or of themselves. Students in physical therapist or physical therapist assistant programs may document when the record is additionally authenticated by the physical therapist or, when permissible by law, documentation by physical therapist assistant students may be authenticated by a physical therapist assistant.

APTA Resources Addressing Documentation

The APTA has a section of its Web page devoted to helping members improve their ability to document. In addition to the previously referenced guidelines and positions, it also contains online continuing education modules on documentation and links to some of the documentation software developed by the APTA. The most important component of that section, however, might be the APTA's **"Defensible Documentation for Patient/Client Management,"** a free 67-page downloadable online tool for members who wish to improve their documentation skills. The introduction to the document cites the following objectives in its development:[15]

- Raising awareness of PTs and PTAs on clinical documentation issues
- Providing usable and clinically relevant information about defensible documentation in patient care
- Identifying legal, regulatory, and payer requirements for clinical documentation
- Providing tools and resources PTs and PTAs need to create documentation that will satisfy all the aforementioned requirements

"Defensible Documentation" uses setting-specific guidelines, case examples, and references to other outside resources to reinforce its suggestions for "best practice" documentation strategies. A summary of this tool is found online in "Defensible Documentation Elements," a two-page outline of tips, strategies, and requirements for writing accurate notes that best support the need for the services provided. In addition, the APTA has also developed checklists to assist clinicians in ensuring that all necessary components of documentation are included in initial examinations, daily notes, and discharge summaries.[15]

FOR REFLECTION

- Make a list of items that you think should be included in every daily progress note. Compare your list with a classmate's, or if possible, to the PTA Visit Note checklist found within "Defensible Documentation Elements" on the APTA website (you must be a member to access this page). How does your list compare?

Common Problems in Documentation

As mentioned, documentation is a skill that must be developed, just like any other. And as occurs with other skills, we sometimes develop bad habits that deviate from best practice performance. The APTA identifies poor legibility as the top reason for payment denials related to documentation. Other documentation problems that lead to denials include the following:[15]

- Incomplete or missing information.
- Use of too many or unfamiliar abbreviations.
- Inconsistency between the services listed as provided and the billing codes used in the charges for those services.

- No reflection of medical necessity for the interventions used or the need for skilled rehabilitation services to deliver them; for example, why does the patient require gait training with physical therapy rather than just being able to walk with nursing staff?
- Repetitious documentation that does not demonstrate progress or change in the patient's status. It is not enough to show that a patient has increased the number of repetitions performed or increased the amount of weight used in a given exercise; the documentation must show how this increase has led to an improved functional status.
- No indication of the time, frequency, and/or duration of interventions used.

In addition, the APTA suggests avoiding use of the phrases "patient tolerated treatment well," "continue per plan," and "as above" within the documentation.[15]

FOR REFLECTION

- When performing documentation, why is the use of the phrases "patient tolerated treatment well," "continue per plan," and "as above" problematic? Identify at least one way that each phrase could be revised to more effectively convey the writer's intent.

SUMMARY

Documentation must accurately reflect the physical therapy services that were provided, why they were necessary, and their effectiveness. By developing a core set of documentation abilities as a student, based on SOAP note concepts and the APTA's guidelines for accuracy, clarity, and content, the PTA will be able to adapt to any format used at a given site. By following these principles and completing only the documentation appropriate for his role, the PTA's documentation will support the delivery of skilled physical therapy services and maximize the potential for appropriate payment for those services.

It cannot be emphasized enough that the ability to document accurately and effectively is as important a skill as any of those that students practice in the classroom. In fact, it may make the difference in advancing in your career. The late Stephen Levine, former APTA Speaker of the House, was an expert in coding and documentation. He expressed a viewpoint common to employers when he stated:

If I, as a private practitioner, have to choose between two therapists to hire—one is a great therapist but can't document and therefore can't get paid for services, and the second is a good therapist who I know can improve his clinical skills but also understands the need to document and do it appropriately—I would go with the latter. I don't think therapists realize that. You have to be able to do it all.[16] (Reprinted with permission from Merion Matters, publishers of ADVANCE Newsmagazines.)

R E F E R E N C E S

1. Wallace J. Technology seduction. *Impact: Private Practice Section of the APTA.* 2015;April:53-55.
2. Venes D, ed. *Taber's Encyclopedic Medical Dictionary.* 22nd ed. Philadelphia, PA: FA Davis; 2013.
3. American Physical Therapy Association. *Guide to Physical Therapist Practice 3.0.* Alexandria, VA: American Physical Therapy Association. http://guidetoptpractice.apta.org/. Updated 2014. Accessed July 6, 2015.
4. American Physical Therapy Association. Guidelines: Physical therapy documentation of patient/client management (BOD G03-05-16-41). http://www.apta.org/uploadedFiles/APTAorg/About_Us/Policies/Practice/DocumentationPatientClientManagement.pdf. Updated 2014. Accessed August 20, 2015.
5. American Physical Therapy Association. Minimum required skills of physical therapist assistant graduates at entry-level. http://www.apta.org/AM/Template.cfm?Section=PTA_Resources1&CONTENTID=53831&TEMPLATE=/CM/ContentDisplay.cfm. Updated 2008. Accessed September 26, 2009.
6. American Physical Therapy Association. *A Normative Model of Physical Therapist Assistant Education: Version 2007.* Alexandria, VA: American Physical Therapy Association; 2007.
7. Hamilton B. *Electronic Health Records.* 3rd ed. New York, NY: McGraw-Hill; 2013.
8. Amatayakul M. *Electronic Health Records: A Practical Guide for Professionals and Organizations.* 4th ed. Chicago, IL: American Health Information Management Association; 2009.
9. American Physical Therapy Association. Support of electronic health record in physical therapy (HOD P06-08-13-11). http://www.apta.org/uploadedFiles/APTAorg/About_Us/Policies/Practice/SupportEHR.pdf. Updated 2012. Accessed August 20, 2015.
10. American Health Information Management Association. Outline of the Medicare and Medicaid program's Electronic Health Record Incentive Program (meaningful use) under the Health Information Technology for Economic and Clinical Health Act (title XIII of the American Recovery and Reinvestment Act of 2009). http://www.ahima.org/downloads/pdfs/advocacy/AHIMA_CMS_Incentive_Program_%28Meaningful_Use%29_Final_Rule_Outline_FINAL_100723.pdf. Updated 2010. Accessed September 12, 2010.
11. Kettenbach G. *Writing Patient/Client Notes: Ensuring Accuracy in Documentation.* 4th ed. Philadelphia, PA: FA Davis; 2009:248.
12. American Physical Therapy Association. Standards of practice for physical therapy (HOD S06-13-22-15). http://www.apta.org/uploadedFiles/APTAorg/About_Us/Policies/Practice/StandardsPractice.pdf. Updated 2013. Accessed August 20, 2015.
13. American Physical Therapy Association. Documentation authority for physical therapy services (HOD P05-07-09-03). http://www.apta.org/uploadedFiles/

APTAorg/About_Us/Policies/Practice/DocumentationAuthority.pdf. Updated 2012. Accessed August 20, 2015.

14. Centers for Medicare & Medicaid Services. CMS manual system transmittal 88: therapy personnel qualifications and policies effective January 1, 2008. http://www.cms.hhs.gov/transmittals/downloads/R88BP.pdf. Updated 2008. Accessed August 14, 2015.

15. American Physical Therapy Association. Defensible documentation for patient/client management. http://www.apta.org/Documentation/DefensibleDocumentation/. Updated 2015. Accessed August 20, 2015.

16. Carter S. Documenting your future. *Adv Phys Therapists & PT Assistants*. 2006;17(8).

Name _____

REVIEW

1. In your own words, briefly describe what type of information should be included in each of the following SOAP note sections:

   Subjective: _____

   Objective: _____

   Assessment: _____

   Plan: _____

2. For each of the following phrases, indicate in which section of the SOAP they would be located by marking each with an *S, O, A,* or *P.*

   _____ Has demonstrated improvement in transfer ability, as amount of assistance needed has decreased.

   _____ Ambulated 75′ × 2 using wheeled walker, required minimal assistance for advancing walker and verbal cueing for proper pattern.

   _____ Patient reports pain in R knee @ 5/10 at rest, 8/10 with activity.

   _____ Nursing reports patient performed independent transfer in bathroom last night.

   _____ Has met weekly goal of independent bed mobility.

   _____ Patient says pain relief lasted for 4 hours after application of electrical stimulation at last intervention session.

   _____ Will ask wife to attend next intervention session to observe and assist with patient's transfers.

   _____ Patient able to go up/down 3 steps w/use of cane and 1 rail; independent with procedure after initial instruction in correct technique.

   _____ Performed AAROM 10 to L knee flexion/extension; patient required total assistance for completing last 10 degrees of motion during final 3 repetitions of extension.

(questions continue on page 160)

_____ May not be ready for d/c to lesser level of care as goal of independent transfers has not been met.

_____ Will ask PT to assess need for joint mobilization techniques to L shoulder.

Application

1. You are on the first day of a clinical experience at a skilled nursing facility and observe one of the PTAs working with a patient who had a right hip replacement because of severe osteoarthritis. The patient is receiving interventions that include ice packs, active assistive range of motion and strengthening exercises, gait training, transfer training, and bed mobility training. The patient's goals include being able to get out of bed independently, transfer independently, and ambulate independently using a wheeled walker within 3 weeks, and to go back to living alone in his home.

Based on the following interventions and topics, list at least two additional questions that the PTA needs to be thinking about to gather enough information to write a comprehensive daily note.

Pain

1. *Where did the patient report feeling pain?*

2.

3.

Gait training

1. *How far did the patient ambulate in today's intervention session?*

2.

3.

Ice packs

1. *To what part of the body were the ice packs applied?*

2.

3.

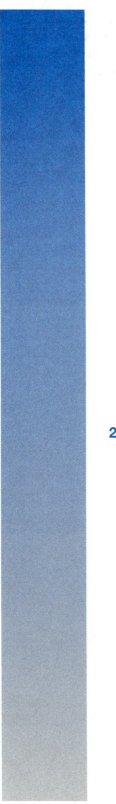

Transfer/bed mobility training

1. *How much assistance did the patient need to go from wheelchair to bed?*

2.

3.

Exercises

1. *What specific exercises were performed today?*

2.

3.

Patient instruction

1. *What specific education was given to the patient today?*

2.

3.

2. Imagine that you have obtained "answers" to each of the questions you listed previously. Organize these answers into the Subjective (S) and Objective (O) sections of a daily progress note:

(S) _____

_____

_____

_____

(O) _____

_____

_____

_____

(questions continue on page 162)

3. Identify at least one possible objective or subjective measure that you could reflect on in the assessment section to demonstrate whether the patient is making improvements in his mobility. Give an example of what you would say about this measure so that it reflects the skilled services this patient needs from PT.

_____

_____

_____

_____

_____

_____

_____

9

The Physical Therapist Assistant and the American Physical Therapy Association

CHAPTER OBJECTIVES

After reading this chapter, the reader will be able to:

- List ways in which the American Physical Therapy Association (APTA) has historically contributed to advancements in physical therapy education and practice.
- Describe the current basic organizational structure of the APTA.
- Describe the evolution of physical therapist assistant (PTA) membership and governance within the APTA.
- Identify APTA core documents and position statements that relate to the PTA.
- Give examples of the ways in which the APTA has developed, defined, and regulated the role of the PTA.
- Describe ways that the APTA is currently supporting the work of the PTA.
- Discuss how the future role of the PTA has been studied by the APTA.
- Identify avenues for PTA involvement in the APTA.
- Recognize the benefits of PTA membership in the APTA.

KEY TERMS AND CONCEPTS

- APTA
- Components: Chapters and sections
- House of Delegates
- Board of Directors
- PTA Caucus
- Student Conclave
- Student Assembly

Miguel *is a newly graduated PTA working in an acute care hospital. During their lunch break, he and two coworkers discuss an article on PTAs that they recently read in* PT in Motion. *Another coworker, Scott, also a PTA, is not familiar with the article and wants to know how Miguel knew about it. Miguel*

(vignette continues on page 164)

replies that he receives the magazine as part of his APTA membership benefits. "I've never really understood what the APTA does," Scott states. He continues, "Besides, why are you a member? Isn't the APTA really just for PTs? Does the APTA really do anything for PTAs?"

QUESTIONS TO CONSIDER

What is the APTA's purpose? How did it evolve? What is the APTA's stance on issues related to the PTA? How can a PTA be involved in the APTA? Why is it important to have PTA representation in the APTA's membership?

Chapter 1 discusses how the PTA position was created through the vision of the **APTA,** the professional organization for physical therapists (PTs), PTAs, and students. This chapter looks at the development of that organization in greater depth, discusses how it has helped regulate and advance the profession in response to changes and challenges in the health-care environment, and considers how it has continued to define and shape the role of the PTA.

The Beginnings of the APTA

By 1920, some physiotherapists or physical therapy technicians (the titles used at that time) were experienced reconstruction aides (see Chapter 1), others were graduates of physiotherapy programs who had not served as reconstruction aides, and still others were physical education program graduates with varying amounts of training in physical therapy modalities.[1] There was a movement to create an organization that would ensure that those working in physical therapy would be following established standards for practice and education. In 1920, about 800 invitations were sent to known physical therapy providers across the country. Those wishing to join this organization were asked to pay $2 for membership and to nominate people to serve in leadership positions. About 120 responses were received. In January 1921, about 30 of those respondents decided to meet in New York City, and the new organization, called the American Women's Physical Therapeutic Association (AWPTA), became official. After that meeting, the 120 members were sent an election ballot, and Mary McMillan, the "first" PT (see Chapter 1), was elected president of the AWPTA. One year later, the name of the organization was changed to the American Physiotherapy Association (APA) to include the small number of men in the profession. Membership struggled to grow during the Great Depression (in 1935 the APA had only 710 members), but by 1946 that number had more than quadrupled. That same year, the APA's name changed to the American Physical Therapy Association to better differentiate the membership from physical therapy physicians, who were now

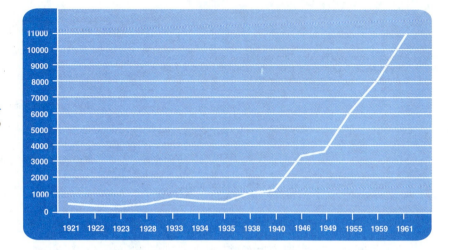

Figure 9-1. APTA Membership 1921–1961.

using the title "physiatrists."[1-3] Figure 9-1 shows the slow but steady increase in APTA membership in the 40 years between 1921 and 1961.

In addition to its initial goal of bringing educational standards into conformity, the purpose of the association quickly evolved to include developing practice standards for PTs (and later for PTAs), promoting advancement of the profession through research and legislation, and advocating for the rights of patients and others in society. Figure 9-2 highlights some of the organization's major milestones throughout the 1900s and into the 2000s.

FOR REFLECTION

■ Review the events listed on the timeline (see Fig. 9-2). If some events are unfamiliar to you, go online to the APTA website (www.apta.org) to find out more about them. Identify one or two events that you consider key to the evolution of the APTA. Why did you pick those events?

The APTA Today

With over 93,000 members (as of January 2016), the APTA currently "seeks to improve the health and quality of life of individuals in society by advancing physical therapist practice, education, and research, and by increasing the awareness and understanding of physical therapy's role in the nation's health care system."[4] Through its advocacy efforts in the areas of health-care practice, policy, and payment systems, the APTA attempts to have a circle of influence that reaches beyond the profession to impact society as a whole. Within the national organization, the APTA also has subdivisions of representation with specific areas of focus and responsibility: component leadership, national leadership, and APTA staff.

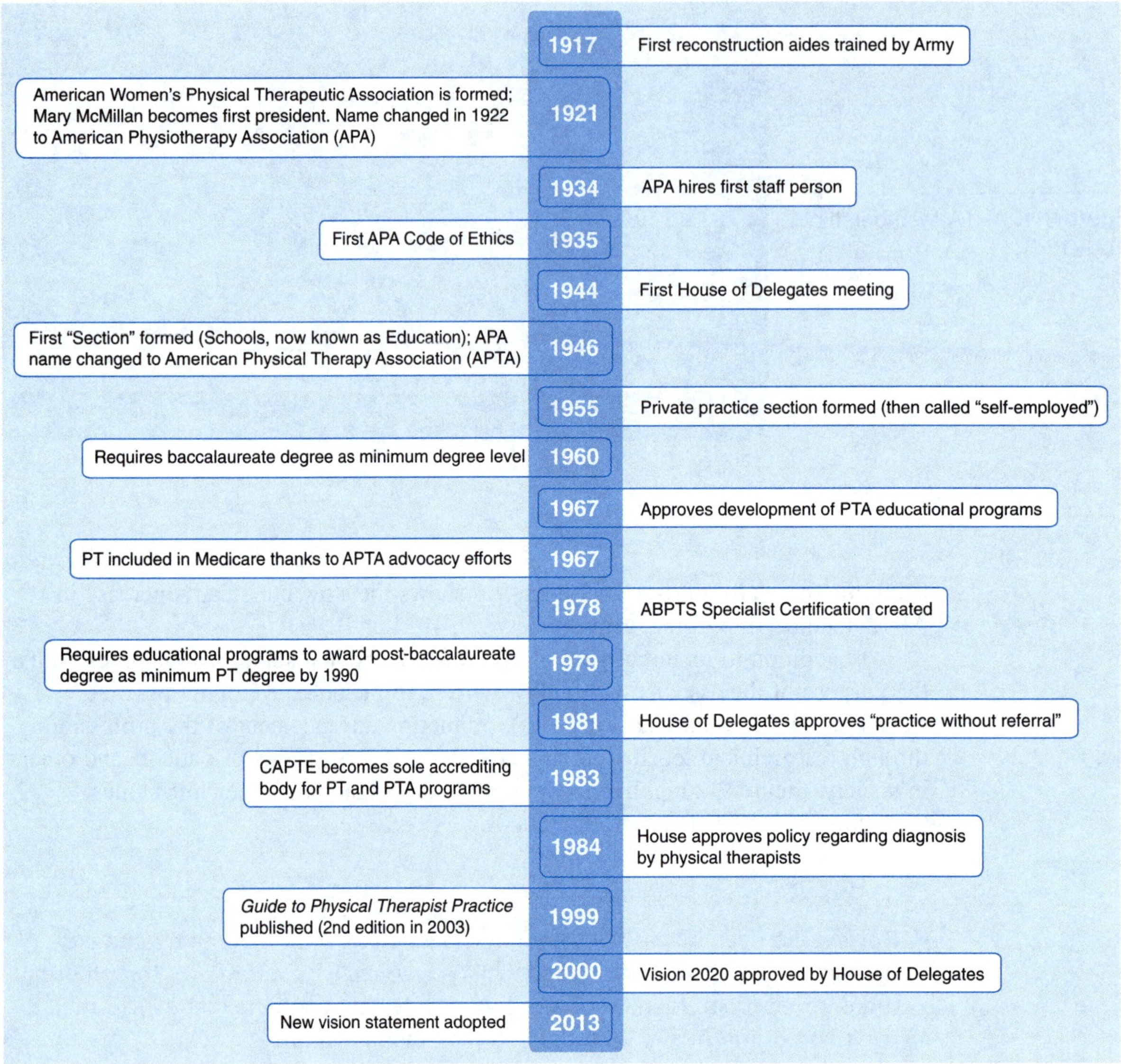

1917	First reconstruction aides trained by Army
American Women's Physical Therapeutic Association is formed; Mary McMillan becomes first president. Name changed in 1922 to American Physiotherapy Association (APA) **1921**	
1934	APA hires first staff person
First APA Code of Ethics **1935**	
1944	First House of Delegates meeting
First "Section" formed (Schools, now known as Education); APA name changed to American Physical Therapy Association (APTA) **1946**	
1955	Private practice section formed (then called "self-employed")
Requires baccalaureate degree as minimum degree level **1960**	
1967	Approves development of PTA educational programs
PT included in Medicare thanks to APTA advocacy efforts **1967**	
1978	ABPTS Specialist Certification created
Requires educational programs to award post-baccalaureate degree as minimum PT degree by 1990 **1979**	
1981	House of Delegates approves "practice without referral"
CAPTE becomes sole accrediting body for PT and PTA programs **1983**	
1984	House approves policy regarding diagnosis by physical therapists
Guide to Physical Therapist Practice published (2nd edition in 2003) **1999**	
2000	Vision 2020 approved by House of Delegates
New vision statement adopted **2013**	

Figure 9-2. Timeline of Highlights in the Evolution of the APTA Through 2015.

Component Leadership: Chapters and Sections

Each state (as well as the District of Columbia) has its own level of APTA membership, called a **chapter.** Membership in the APTA requires a person to join at least one chapter. Most members choose to belong to the chapter located where they live, but some members who live in one state and work in another may choose to be a member in the work state or may even elect to join both chapters. State chapters support and promote national APTA activities and stances; in return, APTA staff members and national leadership support the work of each chapter as it deals with its own issues and needs (such as changes in state legislation that impact physical therapy practice or payment). Many chapters employ an executive director to coordinate the business of the chapter and, depending on the chapter's size, may also have other paid positions to assist the executive director. However, most of the work in chapters is done by those members who volunteer to serve on various committees. Chapters also elect leadership, such as a president, vice president, members of the chapter's board of directors, and representatives to the national APTA House of Delegates (described in the following section). Most chapters host one or two state conferences each year, during which members can participate in continuing education opportunities and receive updates on current practice and legislative issues. Many chapters offer additional continuing education courses throughout the year and promote the profession through involvement in community events and activities.

The **sections** focus on issues and concerns of members working in a particular practice setting, such as acute care, or with a certain patient population or diagnosis, such as pediatrics or oncology. Sections also have presidents and other officers who are elected by the membership of that section. APTA members are not required to join a section, but many members choose to belong to one or more sections that reflect their areas of interest or practice focus. More information on joining a section is presented in Chapter 14.

National Leadership

The APTA's current national governance structure includes the **House of Delegates** and the **Board of Directors.** The House of Delegates is the highest legislative body (see Fig. 9-3). Each chapter elects a predetermined number of voting delegates to

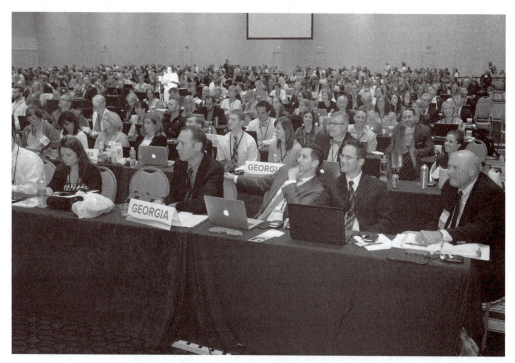

Figure 9-3. Members attending the APTA House of Delegates Meeting, 2015.

represent it within the House of Delegates, based on the number of members in that chapter. In addition, each section elects a member to represent its voice in the House of Delegates, although these representatives are not allowed to vote. The House meets once a year to debate, vote on positions, and elect the Board of Directors. Members of the Board include the association's president and vice president, the speaker and vice speaker of the House, the treasurer, the secretary, and nine at-large Board members. The House gives directives to the Board regarding actions to take and directions in which to lead the association; in return, the Board brings policy suggestions to the House for a vote. The Board of Directors also appoints members to various standing committees, advisory councils, and task forces (short-term work groups), and it is responsible for creating the association's strategic plan and for ensuring that the financial and business dealings of the APTA are handled appropriately. Each director also serves as a liaison to designated chapters and sections, in part to provide assurance to the chapters and sections that their issues are being heard by the Board.

APTA Staff

The APTA also has a number of paid staff positions at its headquarters in Alexandria, Virginia. The Board of Directors appoints a chief executive officer, who oversees the staff activities in addition to working closely with the board to create and shape policy and strategy. APTA staff members take a lead role in legislative issues, support the work of the educational programs, and oversee public relations to promote the profession. Among the APTA departments is one that specifically deals with PTA-related issues, headed by an associate director of PTA services.

Figure 9-4 shows the change in APTA membership from 1987 through 2016.

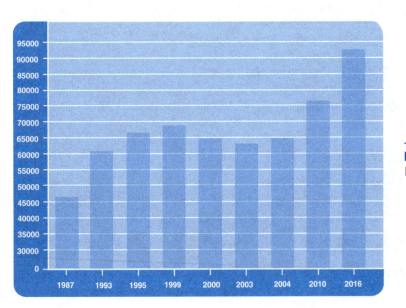

Figure 9-4. Approximate APTA Membership, 1987–2016.

History of PTA Representation Within APTA Governance

From the time the PTA role was created in 1967, there has been controversy within the APTA about PTAs. Establishing the PTA as a formal occupation was not approved by a large margin,[5] and after it was approved, many debates ensued on whether PTAs should become part of the APTA or have their own organization. PTs were divided on this issue. Some worried that having the PTA in the APTA would blur the lines between the two roles and that PTAs would be better served through their own organization. Others believed two separate organizations would be confusing.[6] In 1970, a temporary "affiliate member" category was created for the PTA while a task force took on a 3-year study to investigate the pros and cons of giving PTAs permanent membership status. In 1973, by a margin of one vote, the affiliate category of membership was made permanent.[3] The term "affiliate," which to some indicated something less than full membership, was used to describe the PTA's role in the APTA until that term was formally eliminated in 2005.

Initially, there was no special subgroup in the APTA serving the interests of PTAs. A group of PTA educators created a special interest group (SIG) in the 1970s, but an affiliate SIG was not created until 1983. It took until 1989 before the APTA established the Affiliate Assembly as a new component to which PTAs could belong (at an additional cost). Over time, those active in the Affiliate Assembly realized that PTAs would have a stronger voice if they automatically became part of a PTA subgroup when they became an APTA member. In 1998, a new organizational group called the National Assembly (NA) was formed for PTAs within the APTA. Within the NA, a governance group, the Representative Body of the National Assembly (RBNA) was created. Two of its members were allowed to be nonvoting delegates within the APTA House of Delegates, and the RBNA was allowed to submit motions to the House of Delegates for consideration.[7]

In 2005, a different mechanism for PTA governance was created. The RBNA was dissolved, and the **PTA Caucus** was created by the Board of Directors and approved by the House of Delegates. The PTA Caucus consists of one PTA representative (either elected or appointed) from each APTA chapter. The PTA Caucus meets each year just before the House of Delegates, elects five nonvoting delegates to represent it within the House of Delegates, and has its own designated "community" (a mechanism for year-round electronic communication between caucus members) on the APTA website. The PTA Caucus, like the RBNA before it, is able to bring motions forward to the entire House, and PTA Caucus delegates can address these or any other motions being presented.[8]

Within APTA governance, membership privileges of PTAs differ from those of PTs. For example, only PTs can serve as voting chapter delegates in the House of Delegates; although PTAs can serve as section or PTA Caucus delegates, these are nonvoting positions within the House of Delegates. Only a PT can hold national office, other than those specifically designated for PTAs, but PTAs are allowed to hold many offices at the chapter or section level. When issues come to vote at the chapter or section level, PTAs are allowed to vote, but, until recently, in order to be compliant with APTA bylaws, chapters could count the PTA's vote as only half a vote. However, in response to a motion brought forward by the APTA Board of Directors, the 2015 House of Delegates voted to allow components the right to choose whether they wanted to grant PTAs a full vote.[9] At the time of this writing, multiple states have voted to do so, with additional components planning to vote on this issue in upcoming months.

FOR REFLECTION

- Why do you think some PTs argue against PTAs having a full vote at the chapter and section levels of governance? What could you say to those PTs to counter their arguments?

The APTA'S Influence on the Role of the PTA

Even before the PTA position was created, members of the APTA were already developing the parameters for the PTA's scope of work. As mentioned in Chapter 1, the 1967 proposal to the House of Delegates regarding the formation of the PTA position described the duties that a PTA could perform and the type of supervision that was needed. Subsequent APTA policies and positions have further clarified the utilization of the PTA and the responsibilities of each person in the PT/PTA team. The following standards and positions directly address components of the PTA's role in physical therapist practice:

- Standards of Ethical Conduct for the Physical Therapist Assistant
- Continuing Education for the Physical Therapist Assistant
- Educational Degree Qualification for Physical Therapist Assistants
- Post Entry-Level Education and Recognition of Enhanced Proficiency for the Physical Therapist Assistant
- Physical Therapist and Physical Therapist Assistant License/Regulation
- Consumer Protection Through Licensure of Physical Therapists and Physical Therapist Assistants
- Direction and Supervision of the Physical Therapist Assistant
- Procedural Interventions Exclusively Performed by Physical Therapists
- Provision of Physical Therapy Interventions and Related Tasks
- Supervision of Student Physical Therapist Assistants
- Distinction Between the Physical Therapist and the Physical Therapist Assistant in Physical Therapy
- Levels of Supervision

Many of the APTA's positions regarding the role of the PTA are the result of attempts to clarify the PTA role for clinicians and to reiterate the PT's responsibilities regarding direction and supervision. In doing so, the APTA has taken positions that are considered controversial by some members. An example of one such position, specifically addressing the delivery of interventions, is entitled "Procedural Interventions Exclusively Performed by Physical Therapists" (HOD P06-00-30-36).[10]

Accepted as an official association stance in 2000, this position reiterates that although there are many interventions that PTAs can perform, there are others that they should not. The two interventions singled out in this position are spinal and peripheral joint mobilization/manipulation and sharp selective wound debridement. Many PTs and PTAs disagreed with the House of Delegates' decision to approve this position and believed it was an attempt to "take away" components of interventions in order to restrict the PTA's scope of work. However, the APTA's rationale for excluding these components of intervention from the PTA's scope of work was related to Watts's guidelines for delegation (as reviewed in Chapter 1) and the *Guide*'s components of patient/client management. The complexity of the skills and the ongoing evaluative component required as the skills are being delivered led to the APTA's determination that they were beyond the scope of the PTA's educational preparation and role, even with additional experience and education.

FOR REFLECTION

- Why is it important for APTA members to follow the association's positions, even if they do not always agree with them?

The APTA'S Role in Defining the Future of the PTA

The role of the PT has evolved from being a technician complying with a physician's prescriptive referral to being a primary care provider who independently determines the physical therapy diagnosis and develops the plan of care. As the PT's role has advanced, many PTs and PTAs wondered how those changes would affect the role and utilization of the PTA. The APTA's Vision 2020 mentioned PTAs but gave little insight into how or if they would be used differently. Another APTA document, "Minimum Required Skills of Physical Therapist Assistant Graduates at Entry-Level," identifies the skills expected of any PTA graduate from any educational program. In creating this compilation, other skills were identified that were not currently being fully developed in entry-level clinicians but that were within the scope of the PTA's work. These skills (e.g., leadership, advanced manual soft tissue skills) were identified as ones that would be important for future support of physical therapist practice and would need further development after graduation in order to be performed at the necessary level of competency.[5] A study conducted in the early 2000s supported the need for PTAs to be able to demonstrate the development of their post-graduation advanced skills.[11] These findings led the APTA to create the Recognition of Advanced Proficiency for the Physical Therapist Assistant, a mechanism that, from 2005 to 2016, acknowledged those PTAs who had developed expertise in a specific practice area. After 2016, this recognition will occur through the APTA's Advanced Proficiency Pathways (see Chapter 14).

With the conversion of physical therapist academic programs to the entry-level doctoral degree having occurred much faster than originally anticipated, the differences in the levels of educational preparation for PTs and PTAs have continued to be a topic of discussion within the profession. Many PTs and PTAs believe that the restrictions of an associate degree–level curriculum does not allow PTA educators to deliver entry-level content at an adequate depth or breadth that is required for the PTA graduate to best support physical therapist practice in today's clinical environment. As recently as 2012, the House of Delegates charged the APTA with investigating the need for and feasibility of transitioning the entry-level PTA degree to a bachelor's degree. The results of that study did not conclude that a change was necessary at this time, and therefore the APTA would not move to devote resources to that move. However, it also acknowledged that some programs might have the capability and desire to move forward in this direction, and did not prohibit them from doing so.[12] Currently, a number of PTA programs are investigating the development of entry-level and degree-completion bachelor's programs for PTAs (see Chapter 14).

Opportunities for PTA Involvement and Recognition in the APTA

PTAs have many opportunities to take an active role in the APTA at the chapter level. PTAs can attend state conferences and continuing education workshops alongside PTs. Many chapters and sections also have continuing education opportunities specifically for PTAs at a reduced cost for members. Generally, PTAs are able to participate in most chapter committees and work groups. Most chapters have some type of SIG for PTAs, and some states have PTA positions on their boards of directors. Many states report that it is difficult to recruit PTAs to serve in leadership roles at the chapter level.

PTAs can also be involved in APTA activities at the national level. The APTA website has a specific PTA section that identifies APTA documents and policies that relate to the PTA, along with APTA resources for continuing education and skill development. PTAs can attend one or both of the two APTA conferences that are held annually, the Combined Sections Meeting (usually held in February) and the Annual Conference and Exposition (usually in June). Both of these conferences offer a number of continuing education and networking opportunities, including courses designed specifically for PTAs. Other ways of becoming involved include applying for positions on committees, task forces or work groups seeking PTA representation (through the APTA's online Volunteer Interest Pool), serving as a chapter representative to the PTA Caucus, or running for one of the caucus delegate positions or for the PTA Caucus's Nominating Committee. More information is found in Chapter 14.

Students do not have to wait until graduation before participating in the APTA. For example, APTA offers a student level of membership (the APTA does not differentiate between PT and PTA students), and many chapters have opportunities for students to take part in activities, even if they are not APTA members, at a very minimal cost. On the national level, in addition to attending the previously mentioned conferences, students can participate in the APTA's yearly **Student Conclave.** Students from across the country join APTA leaders to discuss issues related to the profession and have opportunities to participate in mentoring, networking, and career-development activities. Students can also take part in the **Student Assembly,** a governance group that meets at the Student Conclave and sends elected nonvoting representatives to the House of Delegates. In recent years, the Student Assembly has successfully brought a number of motions to the House. Students also serve as ushers at the House of Delegates, helping to keep its operations running smoothly.

Why Be an APTA Member?

The history of interactions between PTs and PTAs within the APTA and its governance systems has not been without controversy. However, the current level of support and inclusiveness for PTAs within the APTA is greater than ever, as can be seen in the many avenues for PTA involvement and skill development within the association. There has never been a better or more important time for PTAs to become APTA members! Ongoing support for the PTA's needs within the APTA and the profession itself can be ensured only if PTAs participate in the organization that has the most influence on their future. Joining the APTA provides PTAs with up-to-date information about practice, payment, and legislative issues; access to the most current clinical evidence; and many educational and networking opportunities. In turn, each individual's membership dues provide additional resources for the association to do its important work. By taking full advantage of APTA membership, every PTA has the opportunity to participate in shaping the association's decisions regarding PTA education and utilization.

FOR REFLECTION

- Return to the scenario at the beginning of this chapter. In your own words, explain to Scott why APTA membership is important for PTAs.

SUMMARY

The APTA is an organization that was initially formed to standardize the profession's educational and practice standards. Its purpose has evolved to include promoting the profession through legislative advocacy and public awareness of health and wellness issues. The APTA has shaped the role of the PTA through position statements and through the evolution of the PTA's ability to participate in association governance. There are many ways for PTAs to be involved in APTA activities on the state and national levels, but the most important mechanism for participation is being a member, as this gives PTAs a voice in shaping the future of the profession.

REFERENCES

1. Moffat M. The history of physical therapy practice in the United States. *J Phys Ther Educ*. 2003;17(3):15-25.

2. Echtermach JL. The political and social issues that have shaped physical therapy education over the decades. *J Phys Ther Educ*. 2003;17(3):26-33.

3. Murphy WB; American Physical Therapy Association. *Healing the Generations: A History of Physical Therapy and the American Physical Therapy Association.* Alexandria, VA: American Physical Therapy Association; 1995:256.

4. American Physical Therapy Association. About us. http://www.apta.org/AboutUs/. Updated 2015. Accessed October 18, 2015.

5. Ward RS. A valuable resource: recent actions confirm the important role of the PTA in the practice of physical therapy and in APTA. *PT Magazine*. 2009;6:14-16.

6. Collopy S, Schenck J, Wood R. Report of three-year study on the physical therapist assistant. *Phys Ther*. 1972;52(12):1300-1307.

7. Wojciechowski M. Celebrating a milestone: 35 years of PTAs. *PT Magazine*. 2004(2):42-49.

8. American Physical Therapy Association. PTA caucus. http://www.apta.org/PTA/Caucus/. Updated 2015. Accessed September 5, 2015.

9. American Physical Therapy Association. Bylaws of the American Physical Therapy Association. http://www.apta.org/uploadedFiles/APTAorg/About_Us/Policies/General/Bylaws.pdf. Updated 2015. Accessed October 18, 2015.

10. American Physical Therapy Association. Procedural interventions exclusively performed by physical therapists (HOD P06-00-30-36). http://www.apta.org/uploadedFiles/APTAorg/About_Us/Policies/Practice/ProceduralInterventions.pdf. Updated 2012. Accessed July 6, 2015.

11. Crosier J. 2008 packet I and background papers: RC 14-08 background paper. http://communities.apta.org/p/do/sd/sid=378&type=0. Updated 2008. Accessed August 20, 2015.

12. American Physical Therapy Association. RC 20-12 feasibility study for transitioning to an entry-level baccalaureate physical therapist assistant degree. *2014 House of Delegates Handbook*. Alexandria, VA: American Physical Therapy Association; 2014:240-241.

Name _____

REVIEW

1. For each of the following decades, list at least one significant event that occurred in the APTA:

1920s: _____

1930s: _____

1940s: _____

1950s: _____

1960s: _____

1970s: _____

1980s: _____

1990s: _____

2000s: _____

2010s: _____

2. Describe the PTA Caucus. Who are its members, what is its purpose, and how is it able to interact with the House of Delegates?

_____

_____

_____

_____

3. Why is it important for PTAs to be members in the APTA?

_____

_____

_____

_____

(questions continue on page 176)

Application

1. Choose one of the APTA position statements listed in this chapter and find out more about it. Why is it important to the PTA? Who is responsible for seeing that it is carried out?

_____

_____

_____

_____

2. What do you believe is the most important purpose of the APTA? Why?

_____

_____

_____

_____

3. There are many opportunities available for you through the APTA. Which ones interest you the most? Why? Describe a way that you will become active in the APTA.

_____

_____

_____

_____

10

Laws Impacting Physical Therapist Practice

CHAPTER OBJECTIVES

After reading this chapter, the reader will be able to:

- Differentiate between a legal and an ethical issue.
- Define various terms used in the legal system.
- Discuss the various formats in which legislation and legal precedent are created.
- Give examples of state and federal laws with specific relevance to health-care providers.
- Discuss principles of law related to health-care malpractice and liability.
- Differentiate between fraud and abuse.
- Explain how power differentials and patient vulnerability influence how certain laws are interpreted in the health-care setting.
- Describe why the nature of physical therapy services may put physical therapists (PTs) and physical therapist assistants (PTAs) at higher risk of having legal complaints filed against them.
- Explain the purpose of the Americans with Disabilities Act.
- Identify mechanisms and resources for minimizing risk while providing physical therapy services.
- Describe the processes of a state licensing agency in dealing with an alleged practice act violation.

KEY TERMS AND CONCEPTS

- Criminal law
- Statutory law
- Civil law
- Common law
- Tort law
- Administrative law
- Negligence
- Health-care malpractice
- Legal duty of care/standard of care
- Fraud

- Abuse
- Assault
- Battery
- Sexual misconduct
- Sexual harassment
- False imprisonment
- Americans with Disabilities Act
- Risk management
- Incident report

Cesar is a PTA working in an outpatient setting. One of the patients on his schedule is Mrs. Johansen, a 75-year-old woman who is receiving interventions to improve the functional use of her right shoulder, which has been impaired by pain related to osteoarthritis. The plan of care includes active and passive stretching to increase the patient's right shoulder range of motion. Cesar has performed the stretches previously without incident. Today, Mrs. Johansen reports that she slipped while getting out of the shower that morning and aggravated her shoulder pain when she caught herself to avoid falling. Cesar notes that Mrs. Johansen's range of motion is the same as it was at her last visit but that it appears to be more guarded. He takes her shoulder up to its end range of motion and encourages Mrs. Johansen to relax. As he applies the stretch, Cesar suddenly senses a slight "give" to the motion. Mrs. Johansen cries out, complains of increased pain, and refuses additional intervention. It is subsequently determined that Mrs. Johansen has sustained a new humeral fracture.*

QUESTIONS TO CONSIDER

What are the laws or legal principles that are relevant to this situation? If Cesar is accused of health-care malpractice, how is any liability determined? Are there actions Cesar took or failed to take that may have increased his liability? Could Cesar's supervising PT potentially be held liable for his actions? What happens if Cesar is accused of a practice act violation?

In previous chapters, this textbook has discussed laws and other regulations unique to physical therapy and supervision of the PTA, and it has reviewed the PT's and PTA's individual and joint responsibilities in adhering to them. However, many other laws and regulations have just as much impact, and they also must be taken into consideration. Some of these laws apply specifically to those working in medical professions; laws in this category are often related to the inherent vulnerability of the patient and the provider's position of power. Others are based on the state and federal statutes and court decisions that dictate the behavior of every person in the community. This chapter discusses the laws and legal principles that, although not unique to physical therapy, direct or influence the delivery of physical therapy services. It also looks at the process in which a state licensing board addresses complaints and reviews the concept of risk management as a way of avoiding potential litigation. Laws related to patient rights, such as those involving consent and confidentiality, are discussed in Chapter 6.

Differentiating Between Legal and Ethical Issues

When someone is accused of an inappropriate action, the issue can be dealt with in as many as four ways, depending on its nature:[1]

- In a criminal court, if a crime has occurred
- In a civil court, if health-care malpractice is involved
- By a licensing board, if a practice act has been violated
- By the professional organization, if the action has violated ethical guidelines

The first three ways of dealing with an inappropriate action are addressed in this chapter. Chapter 5 addresses how ethical beliefs and behaviors, including those mandated by the American Physical Therapy Association (APTA), must be a driving force in decisions and actions. In recent years, it has become increasingly more challenging to distinguish between an ethical and a legal duty in physical therapy.[2,3] One major difference is that the law, in its various forms, applies to everyone in a given society and should take precedence over any decision made on a purely ethical basis. Although something unethical may not be illegal, something illegal is usually unethical.[2] Also, when ethical responsibilities are dictated by way of professional codes or standards, these standards officially apply only to the members of a given professional organization (although it is common for such documents to be used in legal cases against both members and non-members to establish an expected level of appropriate care).[2]

The Law and Physical Therapy

As PTs move toward increased delivery of services in autonomous practice, it is assumed that they will also be held to a higher level of accountability and liability.[4] Even though the PTA's scope of work is unchanged and they remain under the PT's supervision, the potential exists for PTAs to be brought into any lawsuit filed by a patient with whom they have worked. PTAs need to be aware of the types of laws that affect physical therapy so that they better understand their legal responsibilities toward the patient and will work in ways that minimize the chance of being involved in any type of criminal or civil lawsuit. The information in this chapter is designed to provide a general overview of legal standards and concepts and is not in any way meant to represent legal advice. There are several books written by PTs who are also lawyers; for more in-depth information, see the references at the end of this chapter.

Types of Laws

State and federal laws generally fall into three categories. **Criminal law** is that branch of the law that deals with offenses against society. Everyone who lives within a certain jurisdiction is obligated to follow those laws, and when a law is violated, punishment usually follows (jail time, a fine, or both).[5] In criminal law, the defendant must be found guilty "beyond a reasonable doubt"; if measured quantitatively, this is usually thought of as being approximately 90 percent certain that someone is guilty.[4] Criminal law is usually established through **statutory laws** that are enacted by state legislatures or Congress.[6]

Civil laws are those that relate to private offenses, one individual against another, and the punishment for violation of a civil law is usually in the form of monetary damages used to compensate the injured party for being "less than whole."[5] In civil cases, the guilt of the defendant is established (in civil cases usually referred to as being "liable"[5]) by only a "preponderance of the evidence," anything greater than a 50 percent level of confidence of guilt; however, some states require a level of "clear and convincing evidence" (closer to 75 percent) to assign damages.[5] It is possible to be found not guilty of a criminal act but guilty in a civil trial relating to the same series of events.[1] Civil laws are generally established through **common law** (also known as case law), which is determined by a judge's ruling that establishes a precedent (a standing court decision). Common law is considered to be more flexible than statutory law; however, changes in precedents occur only through a ruling by a court at a higher level than the one in which the precedent was established.[6] Another term used to describe civil court actions, especially those having to do with health-care malpractice and personal injury, is **tort law** (the word "tort" comes from Latin for "wrong").[1,3]

The third type of law, **administrative law,** deals with the rules and regulations that apply to government agencies, including those that oversee professions and other fields that provide services to the public. In physical therapy, administrative laws relate to a state's practice act. The organization that regulates physical therapy in a given state, such as a medical board or an independent physical therapy board, determines the type of law under which charges are brought forward when someone is thought to be in violation of a practice act.[4] Health-care professionals are generally thought to have more contact with administrative law representatives and their agencies than any other type of legal division; other examples of administrative law agencies include the Centers for Medicare & Medicaid Services, the Occupational Safety and Health Administration (OSHA), and the Centers for Disease Control and Prevention (CDC).[6]

Although a PTA could be accused of violating laws in any of these categories, the focus in this chapter is on the civil laws related to health-care malpractice and various forms of criminal or civil misconduct that occur as a result of abuse of power.

Health-Care Malpractice

Failing to perform at a minimally acceptable level established to protect the public is called **negligence.** In health care, this is usually referred to as "malpractice." This text uses the term **health-care malpractice** to refer to any action by a health-care provider that results in an adverse outcome and liability on the part of the provider.[1] Civil suits related to health-care malpractice are the most common types of legal issues in which those in the physical therapy profession are involved.[4]

For a claim of health-care malpractice to be substantiated, there are four elements, all of which must be proved to be present. Because health-care malpractice falls under the category of civil law, the level of proof required is that of a preponderance of the evidence (a greater than 50 percent level of confidence that the defendant is guilty).[4] The four elements that must be proved are the following:

- A legal duty of care was owed to the plaintiff
- The legal duty of care was breached or violated
- The breach of duty caused injury to the plaintiff
- The plaintiff suffered recognizable damages[4-6]

Because these criteria are complex and contain legal jargon unfamiliar to most health-care providers (see Table 10-1), they are examined individually in the following sections, as they would be in a court case.

Table 10-1   Legal Terms[1,3–7]

Actual cause	Also known as *sine qua non,* the "but-for" cause: but for this cause, another event could not have occurred
Defendant	The person being prosecuted
Foreseeability	The ability to predict that an event could occur; related to *proximate cause*
Libel	Defamatory (untrue) comments about someone delivered via the written or electronically communicated word
Negligence	Failure to perform at a minimally acceptable level established to protect the public
Plaintiff	The alleged victim in a civil suit
Proximate cause	Also known as legal cause; an event that unforeseeably causes another event to occur—without the first event, the second would not have happened; may or may not be the cause of harm and may limit a defendant's liability
Primary liability	Taking responsibility for one's own actions
Res ipsa loquitur	"The thing speaks for itself"; lessens the burden of proof in a civil case by assuming that something would not have occurred without negligence

(table continues on page 182)

Table 10-1 Legal Terms[1,3–7] **(continued)**

Respondeat superior	"Let the master answer"; see *vicarious liability*
Slander	Defamatory comments about someone delivered via the spoken (or signed) word
Vicarious liability	Responsibility for the actions of someone under one's supervision, such as an employee or volunteer

Was a Legal Duty of Care Owed to the Plaintiff?

A duty is an obligation owed to someone else. In physical therapy, the **legal duty of care** does not usually begin the minute a patient enters a physical therapy clinic. In general, it normally begins at the time the PT examines the patient and establishes that the intervention required is within the PT's scope of practice and level of expertise.[4,8] If the PT determines that the patient's condition and needs are not within the physical therapy scope of practice or the PT's own personal skill set, the duty of care no longer applies.[6]

FOR REFLECTION

- Why is it important to recognize when the duty of care begins? Can you think of a circumstance in which a patient at a clinic might be injured prior to the duty of care having been established?

Was the Legal Duty of Care Breached or Violated?

Having established that a legal duty of care existed, the plaintiff's lawyers must now determine whether it was breached. This could be shown by proving that a PTA committed errors of omission (failing to execute an action that should have been carried out) or performed an inappropriate act (doing something that should not have been done).[5] They must show that the care provided was below the legal **standard of care,** defined as care that would be provided by another "similarly situated" PTA under similar circumstances.[6] In a health-care malpractice case, expert witnesses are generally brought in to establish the current standard of care—generally considered to be the minimally acceptable level of practice[5]—that should have been provided in the situation under debate.[2]

Did the Breach of Duty Cause Injury to the Plaintiff?

Sometimes a breach of duty is not the actual cause of an injury. Causes assigned to an injury may be "actual" or "proximate." If the injury is determined to be related to a proximate cause, one that was unforeseeable (unpredictable), the defendant may not be considered liable, even though care may still have been breached.[1] For example, if a patient sustains a fractured hip during a transfer, undergoes surgery to repair it, and in the process is found to have a cancerous tumor within the bone, the injury might be considered to have occurred because of proximate cause, even if a breach of duty (such as not using a transfer belt) occurred during the transfer.

Did the Plaintiff Suffer Recognizable Damages?

Lawyers must be able to prove that the plaintiff suffered damages. In legal terms, damages are losses that require compensation. Examples include economic losses such as a loss of income from being unable to work, but also can include noneconomic losses such as pain and suffering, disfigurement, and so on. Lawyers must be able to prove that the plaintiff suffered damages and should be awarded compensation <AU1> in order to help the plaintiff recover from these losses. Even if some breach of care occurred (such as a patient sustaining a fall), if there are no losses connected with the incident (the patient is able to move without pain, resumes normal activities), a claim of health-care malpractice may not be upheld. Conversely, if losses occurred because of behavior on the part of the defendant that appears to have been reckless and without regard for others, monetary punitive damages may be awarded to punish the defendant and, it is hoped, prevent others from doing the same thing.[4]

FOR REFLECTION

- Go back to the scenario at the beginning of this chapter. If Mrs. Johansen filed a claim of health-care malpractice against Cesar, do you think it would stand up against these four criteria? Which ones might be easier to prove than the others? Why?

Legal Responsibility Within the PT/PTA Team

Each member of the PT/PTA team is responsible for knowing the laws that apply to him and his workplace and each retains individual responsibility for following them, a legal principle referred to as primary liability.[9] A PTA is responsible for knowing the constraints of his state's practice act, and if directed to perform an act that is outside his scope of work or illegal in some other way, he is responsible for refusing to perform such an action. In other words, saying, "The PT told me to do it" will never excuse a PTA's actions. In cases in which a PTA has some knowledge of inappropriate behavior on the part of the PT but fails to report this behavior to the proper authorities, the PTA may not hold the same level of responsibility for the action itself but may face sanctions for his failure to act.[10]

The situation is a bit different for the PT. Because the PTA works under the direction and supervision of the PT, the PT retains ultimate responsibility for any actions that the PTA performs.[4] One legal principle that applies to this situation is called "vicarious liability," in which a supervisor (or employer) is legally and financially responsible for the actions of those he supervises. Another term for this concept is *respondeat superior,* Latin for "let the master answer."[1] Even though the supervision provided might not be on site (as allowed by law), the responsibility for appropriate supervision remains with the PT. Therefore, in situations in which the PTA is held liable for health-care malpractice, the PT may also be held liable. A PTA who performs a deliberate act of assault or battery (defined in the next section), such as brandishing a weapon in the workplace or committing sexual misconduct, is an example of a situation in which a PT is unlikely to be held liable for the actions of a PTA.[6]

Laws Related to Abuse of Power

Because of the power advantage that providers hold in the patient/provider relationship, a number of laws are designed to protect the patient. In addition, other laws that relate to all of society (criminal laws) can take on a different connotation when applied to the unique relationships that develop between patients and their caregivers. Some of the laws related to patient rights (such as the Health Insurance Portability and Accountability Act, informed consent, and advance directives) are addressed in Chapter 6. The following is a nonexclusive description of types of legal wrongdoing that may result in civil, criminal, or administrative action being taken against a physical therapy clinician.

Fraud

Accusations of **fraud** can happen when someone is suspected of having knowingly misrepresented the truth or concealed facts to the detriment of another.[4] Instances in which fraud has been known to have occurred in health care include intentionally billing for services not provided, billing for services provided by unqualified providers, or making a patient referral for services at a clinic in which the referring person has a financial interest.[1,4] Fraud is paired with the term **abuse.** Abuse as used in legal texts more often refers to physical abuse. However, when used in connection with the word "fraud," it generally implies some type of "misuse"[11] that has occurred (usually unintentionally), such as using an inappropriate billing code for a service provided or billing for services that are determined to be not medically necessary.[3] As a PTA, being directed to bill in a fraudulent manner or using a billing code in a way that one does not know is fraudulent does not mean that the PTA is without guilt; as is often stated, *ignorance of the law is no excuse.*[4]

Circumstances in which a physical therapy provider might be accused of committing physical abuse is addressed in the section discussing "assault and battery."

Failure to Report Suspected Physical Abuse

In most states, health-care providers are legally required to report suspected child, domestic, or elder abuse[1,11] and have an ethical obligation to do so as well.[10,12] Failure to report suspected abuse may be considered a breach of duty and could result in the clinician being served with a claim of health-care malpractice and/or having a complaint filed with the appropriate licensing board.[1,4] Any suspected abuse should first be reported to the supervising PT, who can help the PTA report it to the proper authorities. In addition, the circumstances leading to the questioning of abuse (such as physical signs or unusual behaviors and/or comments from the patient or caregivers) should be documented as objectively as possible. The clinician's role is not to prove that abuse has occurred but rather to report the signs and symptoms of possible abuse.[4]

FOR REFLECTION

FOR REFLECTION

- According to Scott, physical abuse is frequently underreported by clinicians.[1] Why do you think that is the case?

Assault and Battery

"Assault" and "battery" are terms that are frequently linked together, but they have separate meanings.[9] **Assault** is the fear or anticipation of being harmed through the application of force or unwanted physical contact. The actual impermissible application of that physical contact or force is considered **battery**.[1,4,5,11] An accusation of assault and/or battery can be dealt with as either a criminal or civil claim: because of the lesser level of proof needed in civil lawsuits, it is often easier to "prove" in a civil court.[4] Because of the nature of frequent physical contact often required during the delivery of physical therapy services, sometimes close to intimate parts of the body, clinicians need to be especially cautious and proactive to avoid any accusation of assault and/or battery. They must clearly explain how they are going to expose or touch a patient, explain why the touch or exposure is necessary, and obtain permission for any touch used on a patient, all before proceeding. Facilities may also consider having policies that allow patients to have a chaperone (usually of the same gender) present during any treatment that might be applied to or expose intimate parts of the body or that will be performed in a private room.[4,11]

Sexual Misconduct and Sexual Harassment

Once again, two terms are connected but have different meanings. **Sexual misconduct** is *any* sexual contact, sexual assault, or sexual battery between a patient and a health-care provider. As with assault and battery, because of the frequent hands-on contact involved in the profession, PTs and PTAs may be at greater risk of sexual misconduct accusations than other health-care providers.[8] Even a relationship that both parties claim is consensual should be considered sexual misconduct, as most experts feel that it is impossible for a clinician to have a consensual relationship with a patient/client.[8] Because of the imbalance of power in the patient/provider relationship, the vulnerability of patients, and the special duty of trustworthiness that providers are to uphold with their clients, Scott maintains that "any sexual relationship between a professional and client is inherently potentially exploitative, and therefore to be avoided at all costs."[1] The Code of Ethics and the Standards of Ethical Conduct also prohibit any exploitative relationships and any sexual relationships with patients/clients.[10,12] The question is sometimes asked whether, after a given period, it is ethically permissible to have a sexual relationship with a former patient. Susan Sisola, a former member of the APTA's Ethics and Judicial Committee (EJC), has written:

> The patient's vulnerability is not something that can be assumed to dissipate immediately at the end of the final treatment session. ... The EJC does not believe that any arbitrary period of time (e.g. 3 months or two years) can answer whether initiation of a romantic or sexual relationship with a former patient would be ethical. ... The determination ... depends not on a quantifiable passage of time ... but rather on a host of qualitative circumstances relating to the patient, the physical therapist, and the relationship between them. Any significant disparity between the power, status, and emotional vulnerability of the former patient and that of his or her PT strongly suggest the potential for an exploitive relationship.[13]

Although Sisola's words single out the PT, this author assumes that the EJC's opinion likewise applies to the PTA.

Sexual harassment is different from sexual misconduct. It is not between the patient and the provider but between employees in the workplace. **Sexual harassment** is defined as unwelcome verbal or physical conduct of a sexual nature that:

- Implies that submitting to it must occur as a condition of employment or employment decisions (in legal terms this is referred to as *quid pro quo,* meaning "this for that"[3]), or
- Causes unreasonable interference with one's work performance or creates an intimidating, hostile, or offensive work environment.[1,8]

Whereas sexual misconduct claims can often be heard in criminal court (as well as in civil courts and in front of administrative boards), sexual harassment is generally a civil wrong.[11] Whereas making one's workplace a nonthreatening environment is every employee's responsibility, managers and other administrative personnel have primary responsibility for doing so and can be held accountable if they fail to take action on an employee's complaint that is eventually substantiated.[1]

An allegation of sexual misconduct or sexual harassment, even if eventually disproved, can be detrimental to one's career. In addition, professional liability insurance often does not provide coverage for claims related to these types of wrongs.[8]

FOR REFLECTION

- According to one national survey, a majority of PTs reported having worked with patients who exhibited inappropriate sexual behaviors.[14] Should this be considered sexual misconduct? Should it be considered sexual harassment? Defend your answer.

False Imprisonment

In health care, **false imprisonment** means something different from that which might occur in the prison system. In physical therapy, a clinician could be accused of false imprisonment any time he intentionally does something to unlawfully restrict a patient's movement. This could include acts such as refusing to let a patient discharge himself from a facility against medical advice, or attempting to prevent a patient from leaving the clinic until he has paid an overdue bill for services. A charge of false imprisonment is a type of civil tort called an "intentional tort"; as the name implies, this means that the perpetrator intentionally committed a given wrongful act.[1,5]

Other Legal Considerations in Physical Therapist Practice

Americans with Disabilities Act Requirements

The Americans with Disabilities Act of 1990 (ADA) is a federal law established to prevent discrimination based on a person's disability. In order to qualify under the ADA as having a disability, a person must show that she has "a physical or mental impairment that substantially limits one or more major life activities; a record of such an impairment, or being regarded as having such an impairment."[15] The law is designed to allow persons with disabilities equal access to employment. If a person with a disability cannot perform the essential functions of a job, but can do so if provided with "reasonable accommodations," these accommodations must be provided by the employer, unless doing so would be an "undue hardship" for that employer.[6,15] If an employee lacks proper identification and documentation of a disability, an employer is not obligated to provide an accommodation. However, many employers are very supportive of the ADA and work proactively with employees to determine appropriate accommodations; physical therapy may be used in a consultative role to assist in these determinations.[6]

As employees in the workplace, PTs and PTAs have rights under the ADA and should not hesitate to report disabilities that interfere with the performance of their employment duties. Likewise, physical therapy students also are protected under the ADA. Many physical therapy programs ask students to read a document that describes the essential functions of the classroom and clinical environments, and then sign a form stating that they are able to perform these functions.[16] If they require an accommodation to perform those functions, they are generally required to obtain medical documentation of their disability and must work through a department within the academic institution that specializes in services for students with disabilities, to determine and obtain the appropriate accommodation. Students are encouraged to be proactive in identifying known or suspected disabilities, as doing so may make a student with a disability more likely to be successful in school.[16] However, academic programs are not responsible for making accommodations for disabilities that are not formally reported to them.[6]

Risk Management

Avoiding allegations of illegal behavior is a component of **risk management.** The broad goals of a risk management program are maximizing the quality of care provided so that no injuries occur while at the same time minimizing financial loss.[3,11] It can be challenging for an organization to do both simultaneously, especially in this era of managed care, which appears to some to be focused more on cost-control than on the quality of the care provided.[5]

In health care, risk management is often approached in an interdisciplinary manner, with upper-level administration being ultimately accountable.[3,5,11] At the same time, effective risk management can occur only if each individual is responsible for providing optimal patient care while following established facility procedures, legal regulations, and professional standards of ethical behavior.

FOR REFLECTION

- In the opening scenario, what actions could Cesar have taken to demonstrate his awareness of risk management principles?

One of the best ways of minimizing risk is to maintain thorough and accurate documentation records on all patients. Nicholson states that a jury in a physical therapy malpractice case is likely to hear a version of the adage that states, "If it wasn't documented, it wasn't done."[4] The principles of effective documentation on a day-to-day basis are addressed in Chapter 8. Scott maintains that "the documentation of clinical patient care activities is as important as the rendition of care itself."[5] In addition to being a "best practice" standard, having thorough documentation may be crucial to a clinician's defense if an accusation of health-care malpractice is filed.[4,5] A PT and PTA should meticulously document when the patient's response to an intervention is atypical or if anything unusual is noted through observation or palpation. If any type of unusual event occurs in therapy (a fall, a skin tear, even an unusual verbal exchange), an **incident report** should be completed by the person observing or discovering the event. An incident report is a separate document describing something out of the ordinary that happens. It may vary in format from facility to facility, but it is usually written in an objective narrative format and is kept with departmental records, not in the patient's chart.[3] Incident reports can be used for noting areas in need of quality improvement or immediate corrective action to ensure patient safety, but they should also be thought of as a way to ensure accurate recall of an event in case of future legal action.[5] Incident reports are probably not completed as often as they should be, possibly because of clinicians' fear that the report may be used against them in court.[5,11] However, if completed "in anticipation of litigation," incident reports are protected documents that do not need to be shared with a prosecuting legal team.[4]

Many pages on the APTA's website provide extensive information on other risk management strategies.[17] One way to minimize potential financial risk is to obtain professional liability insurance. Academic institutions are required to have liability insurance for students who participate in clinical experiences, and many clinicians have some type of liability insurance through their employers. One benefit to a clinician having his own liability insurance, in addition to having greater financial coverage for a claim (which minimizes the risk for out-of-pocket costs),[4] is that it typically provides legal counsel for the individual involved. This may be advantageous, as the legal counsel provided by the facility may not be focusing solely on the interests of the individual employee.[5] It is interesting to note that the same amount of liability insurance is much less expensive for physical therapy practitioners than it is for physicians, an indication of the low risk associated with the profession.[8] However, as more and more PTs work under a model of autonomous practice, the level of exposure to risk is expected to rise.[4]

The State's Role in Handling Accusations of Practice Act Violations

The role of the state licensing board (or comparable state agency) is to protect the public by ensuring that those in the profession for which it has oversight are practicing at a standard level of competency. It is the clinician's responsibility to demonstrate competency for initial licensure or license renewal in whatever manner prescribed by that agency. However, when a complaint is filed against a clinician, the state agency is responsible to determine whether patient safety is at risk because of a lack of competency and/or if the practice act has been violated.[1,4]

Filing an administrative complaint against a clinician is a formal process with strict criteria. In some court cases, complaints have been dismissed, not because the clinician was found to be innocent but because the complainant (the person filing the complaint) did not follow proper procedure.[4] In most states, a complaint must be filed in writing, sometimes on a special form that must be notarized. The complainant can usually remain anonymous if he chooses to do so. However, complainants may be informed that investigating the complaint can be done more thoroughly if the clinician in question is able to respond to the specific incident, which can occur only if the patient's identity is revealed.[18]

When a formal complaint is filed, the state board then does a preliminary "probable cause" hearing, in which the complaint is reviewed, and the evidence for or against the complaint is examined. If there is no identification of probable cause, the complaint is dismissed and remains confidential. The complainant can then choose to appeal the decision, drop the matter, or file a civil lawsuit. If, however, the state board determines that there is probable cause that a violation occurred, another hearing is scheduled. At this point, the complaint would become part of the public record. If, in the subsequent hearing, the board decides that the practice act has been violated, it will issue some type of sanction against the clinician. Sanctions may include receiving a written reprimand, being assigned remedial course work to demonstrate competency, receiving a fine, being suspended, or having a license permanently revoked (canceled).[1,4]

The role of a state physical therapy association chapter is often confused with that of a state licensing board. The state chapter does not have the authority to discipline clinicians for legal violations, as does the state licensing board, but it can issue sanctions for ethical violations, a process that is described in Chapter 5.

S U M M A R Y

Having an awareness of the laws pertaining to health care is essential in today's litigious society. By understanding how legal concepts apply to the delivery of PT services and by developing a greater sensitivity to the unique vulnerability of the physical therapy patient, PTAs can provide physical therapy in a manner that correctly follows legal statute and precedent, minimizes their own personal risk of liability, and maximizes the safety of the patient and the integrity of the patient-practitioner relationship.

R E F E R E N C E S

1. Scott RW. *Promoting Legal Awareness in Physical and Occupational Therapy.* St. Louis, MO: Mosby; 1997:310.
2. Scott RW. Supporting professional development: understanding the interplay between health law and professional ethics. *J Phys Ther Educ*. 2000;14(3): 17-19.
3. Swisher LL, Krueger-Brophy C. *Legal and Ethical Issues in Physical Therapy.* Boston, MA: Butterworth-Heinemann; 1998:231.
4. Nicholson S. *The Physical Therapist's Business Practice and Legal Guide.* Sudbury, MA: Jones & Bartlett; 2008:399.
5. Scott RW. *Health Care Malpractice: A Primer on Legal Issues for Professionals.* 2nd ed. New York, NY: McGraw-Hill; 1999.
6. Scott R. *Promoting Legal and Ethical Awareness: A Primer for Health Professionals and Patients.* Philadelphia, PA: Mosby Elsevier; 2009:273.
7. Scott RW, Petrosino C, Cooperman J. *Physical Therapy Management.* St. Louis, MO: Mosby/Elsevier; 2008:226.
8. Cooperman J. Legal and ethical management issues. In: Scott RW, Petrosino CL. *Physical Therapy Management.* St. Louis, MO: Mosby Elsevier; 2008:102-145.
9. Scott RW. *Foundations of Physical Therapy.* New York, NY: McGraw-Hill; 2002:484.
10. American Physical Therapy Association. Standards of ethical conduct for the physical therapist assistant. http://www.apta.org/uploadedFiles/APTAorg/About _Us/Policies/Ethics/StandardsEthicalConductPTA.pdf. Updated 2015. Accessed August 13, 2015.
11. Nosse LJ, Friberg DG, Kovacek PR. *Managerial and Supervisory Principles for Physical Therapists.* 2nd ed. Baltimore, MD: Lippincott Williams & Wilkins; 2005.
12. American Physical Therapy Association. Code of ethics for the physical therapist. http://www.apta.org/uploadedFiles/APTAorg/About_Us/Policies/Ethics/ CodeofEthics.pdf. Updated 2009. Accessed August 22, 2015.
13. Sisola SW. Patient vulnerability: ethical considerations for physical therapists. *PT Magazine*. 2003;11(7):46-50.

14. deMayo R. Patient sexual behaviors and sexual harassment: a national survey of physical therapists. *Phys Ther*. 1997;77:739-744.

15. U.S. Department of Justice. Information and technical assistance on the Americans with Disabilities Act. http://www.ada.gov/. Updated 2015. Accessed September 7, 2015.

16. Rangel A, Wittry A, Boucher B, Sanders B. A survey of essential functions and reasonable accommodations in physical therapist education programs. *J Phys Ther Educ*. 2001;15(1):11.

17. American Physical Therapy Association. Risk management. http://www.apta.org/RiskManagement/. Updated 2012. Accessed August 22, 2015.

18. Minnesota Board of Physical Therapy. Complaint review process: questions and answers. http://mn.gov/health-licensing-boards/images/Questions%2520and%2520Answers%2520about%2520the%2520Board.pdf. Updated 2013. Accessed August 22, 2015.

Name _____

REVIEW

1. List and explain the four elements that must be proved to substantiate a claim of health-care malpractice.

   _____

   _____

   _____

   _____

2. Compare and contrast each of the following pairs of terms:

   a. Statutory law/common law: _____

   _____

   _____

   b. Criminal law/civil law: _____

   _____

   _____

   c. Fraud/abuse: _____

   _____

   _____

   d. Assault/battery: _____

   _____

   _____

   e. Sexual misconduct/sexual harassment: _____

   _____

   _____

(questions continue on page 194)

Application

1. In the following situations, state the likelihood that a claim of negligence could be substantiated. Do you have enough information to make this determination? If so, identify the person or persons whom you think might be held liable. If not, determine the additional information that you might need to make a decision.

A. A patient has had recent surgery to repair a torn rotator cuff. The PT instructs the PTA to progress the exercises "as tolerated," and the PTA has the patient start exercises using resistance. When the patient returns to the physician for a follow-up examination, the physician informs him that the repair does not appear to have been successful.

_____

_____

_____

_____

B. A patient has sustained a hip fracture and is not allowed to bear weight through the involved lower extremity, but he has difficulty maintaining his non-weight-bearing status during activity. While ambulating in physical therapy, he frequently puts his full weight on his involved leg despite being reminded not to do so. The patient later needs a hip replacement as a result of the fracture not healing properly.

_____

_____

_____

_____

C. A patient performing stabilization exercises on a ball falls to the ground and breaks a wrist when the ball suddenly ruptures.

_____

_____

_____

_____

D. A patient in the clinic parking lot slips and falls, hitting his head and sustaining a cut that requires stitches.

_____

_____

_____

_____

2. For each of the following behaviors, identify the law that a PT or PTA might be accused of violating:

■ Telling a patient, "If you don't help more when I transfer you, I'm going to drop you!"

_____

_____

_____

_____

■ Restraining a patient in a wheelchair without proper medical orders.

_____

_____

_____

_____

■ Exposing a client's buttocks without permission or a rationale for doing so.

_____

_____

_____

_____

(questions continue on page 196)

- Using excessive force in performing a patient's range of motion exercises.

_____

_____

_____

_____

11

Payment for Physical Therapist Services

CHAPTER OBJECTIVES

After reading this chapter, the reader will be able to:

- Describe the evolution of the ways patients have paid for health-care services.
- Discuss trends in the current health-care environment and their impact on payment.
- Differentiate among Medicare Part A, Medicare Part B, and Medicaid.
- Describe the main coding systems that are used in requesting payment for physical therapist services.
- Identify factors that are used to determine annual payment code rates.
- Give examples of site-specific Medicare outcome measure requirements.
- Discuss the new outcomes database and payment system currently being developed by American Physical Therapy Association (APTA).
- Give examples of new payment models being driven by the Patient Protection and Affordable Care Act.
- Discuss the APTA's advocacy efforts related to payment and health-care reform.

KEY TERMS AND CONCEPTS

- Third-party payer
- Managed care
- Health maintenance organization
- Preferred provider organization
- Copayment
- Deductible
- Triple aim
- Patient Protection and Affordable Care Act
- Prior authorization
- Centers for Medicare & Medicaid Services
- Medicare A and B
- Medicaid
- International Classification of Diseases (ICD) codes
- Current Procedural Terminology (CPT) codes
- Resource-Based Relative Value Scale
- Physician Fee Schedule
- Fee for service
- Diagnosis-related groups
- Prospective payment system
- Outcomes and Assessment and Information Set
- Resource Utilization Groups
- Case Mix
- Minimum Data Set
- G-codes
- Physician Quality Reporting System

- Accountable care organizations
- Legislative Action Center
- Integrity in Practice campaign
- Physical Therapy Classification and Payment System
- PTeam/Key Contact

E*nrique and Taylor have just returned to classes after having completed their first full-time clinical experiences. Enrique, who was at a subacute facility, brings up the topic of billing. "It was challenging for me to keep track of the minutes of therapy I provided, and so hard to make sure we met the patient's RUG levels," he comments. Taylor, whose clinical was at an outpatient clinic, looks confused, and says, "What is a RUG level? I don't remember talking about that when we did our billing. But the PTs at my clinic spent a lot of time tracking G-codes and outcome measures for PQRS." Enrique shakes his head and says, "I know the RUG levels had something to do with the minutes we documented on the MDS." Taylor has no idea what Enrique is talking about and wonders, "Why were we doing things so differently? Was my clinic doing something wrong?"*

QUESTIONS TO CONSIDER:

How has payment for health-care services evolved over time? What factors determine how billing for payment for physical therapist services is done? How do billing requirements vary based on type of facility? How does a patient's insurance coverage impact how billing is performed and payment is received? What other factors influence payment for physical therapy? What is the APTA doing to ensure that physical therapy clinics are fairly compensated for services provided and to prevent fraudulent billing practices?

In addition to being able to accurately document the services one delivers during an intervention session, as described in Chapter 8, physical therapist assistants (PTAs) must also be able to accurately submit charges for those interventions in a manner that will ensure payment for them. As health-care systems have evolved, payment mechanisms have become more complicated. This chapter addresses the ways that payment for physical therapy is determined, and how the format for billing and the amount of payment received may vary based on the setting in which the service is provided. It also reviews how the APTA works to ensure that physical therapists (PTs) and PTAs receive fair payment for the services they provide, and looks at its efforts to combat fraud and abuse in payment submissions.

The Evolution of Payment for Health-Care Services

The ways in which providers have been compensated for their services have changed considerably over the years. In previous centuries, physicians often traded their services for goods or services provided by the patient. For example, a farmer might have given a doctor some chickens the family had raised in payment for assisting with the birth of a child. There was no type of health insurance for patients until the late 1800s, and those plans primarily provided for income lost during a patient's illness or, in case of death, covered funeral costs.[1] However, the Depression of 1929 caused widespread financial difficulties for patients and hospitals alike. A plan covering hospital costs was developed that year by Baylor University Hospital for its employees; this later evolved into the country's first Blue Cross plan.[1,2] The first Blue Shield plan, covering physician fees, was developed by the California Medical Association in 1939, but the two plans did not merge until the mid-1970s.[2] Blue Cross/Blue Shield is an example of a **third-party payer,** an organization or agency that pays some or all of the costs of services provided to patients.[3]

In the mid-1930s, there was legislative discussion about creating a system of mandatory health-care insurance for everyone in the United States, similar to that which had been developed in European countries. However, the American Medical Association strongly opposed this action, fearing that it would threaten its ability to practice independently. By the 1940s, employer-paid health insurance was commonplace, and this also diffused the momentum toward government-provided insurance.[1,2] It was not until the late 1950s that the idea of government-provided insurance began to be reconsidered, specifically for the elderly and impoverished. There was now a critical mass of elderly people, many of whom were in greater need of health-care services than the younger population, but who were ineligible for employer-based coverage and could not afford private coverage. In 1965, the government adopted Medicare Parts A and B to provide hospital and medical coverage for older adults (which soon after included physical therapy, as noted in Chapter 1). At that time, the government also initiated the Medicaid program for those with lower incomes.[2] Both Medicare and Medicaid are addressed in greater detail later in this chapter.

The latter part of the 20th century saw huge advances in medical care, and the costs associated with those services continued to rise. This contributed to the development of **managed care** organizations that propose to keep costs down by avoiding duplication of services and coordinating the delivery of care.[1] The first managed care systems were called **health maintenance organizations** (HMOs). HMOs attempt to control the costs of their enrollees' care by restricting patients' choices of providers, focusing on preventive care, and decreasing the use of specialists and hospitalization.[3] However, patient satisfaction with the HMO model initially was low because of the restrictions in one's choice of providers and negative perceptions about the quality of care received.[1] Subsequently, another type of managed care model was developed, the **preferred provider organization** (PPO). In the PPO model, patients are allowed greater choice in providers but are incentivized to use the providers within that network, with higher copayments/out-of-pocket costs incurred with the use of nonpreferred or "out of network" providers.[1,3] Most private (i.e., not government funded) health-care insurance today is provided under some type of managed care format (e.g., HMO or PPO).[1] Variations in coverage can include the patient's responsibilities for the monthly out-of-pocket premium (policy cost), the **copayment** charge (the amount or percentage that the patient must pay for a given office visit or prescription), and the policy **deductible** (the amount that the patient must pay before insurance payment begins).[3]

Despite the use of managed care and several attempts by the U.S. Congress to legislate improved payment systems,[2] health-care costs in the United States and the numbers of those either unable to afford or access health insurance have continued to rise in the 21st century.[4] Full exploration of the reasons for these increases is beyond the scope of this textbook, but contributing factors for the rising costs of health-care have been blamed on the aging of our population coupled with greater life expectancy (and therefore greater utilization of health-care services), excessive ordering of expensive diagnostic procedures in an attempt to defray the costs of the diagnostic equipment, inefficiency and duplication of services, increased pharmaceutical costs, and general overuse of medical tests and referrals to specialty providers because of fear of malpractice lawsuits.[1,2,5] The reasons for the increase in the number of uninsured are thought to include (but certainly may not be limited to) higher unemployment rates, fewer employers providing health insurance, and higher costs of employees' out-of-pocket contributions toward employer-provided plans.[3] Lack of insurance often means that individuals end up in an emergency room (ER) for primary care because of federal regulations that say they cannot be turned away in that setting owing to lack of funds.[2] Costs for services in the ER are often higher than they would be in a physician's office, and often end up being written off by hospitals when individuals cannot pay for the charges incurred. Some of these costs then are passed on to all consumers through higher charges for services in general.[1,2] By the late 2000s, all of these factors contributed to an even greater outcry for health-care reform that became focused on the **triple aim**: decreasing costs, improving health, and making the individual patient's perception of his health-care experience a more positive one.[6]

In 2010, after months of debate, Congress passed the **Patient Protection and Affordable Care Act,** more commonly called the Affordable Care Act (ACA). Immediately after the law was passed, multiple states joined a federal lawsuit challenging its requirements for Medicaid expansion and mandated individual coverage, but in 2013, the Supreme Court upheld the ACA's constitutionality.[1] It is believed that the ACA will have more impact than any other legislation since the inception of Medicare and Medicaid, affecting everyone in the United States.[3] The ACA is more than 900 pages long and its complex requirements are being clarified, refined, and implemented gradually over a period of years, with some mandates not having to be in place until 2019.[1] The APTA has broken down the complexity of the new regulations into four major areas of impact for physical therapy providers:[7]

• Improved health insurance coverage for individuals through Medicaid expansion, increased requirements for employers to provide insurance options, and the creation of health-care "marketplaces" in which individuals are required to purchase insurance if unavailable through other means. As of 2014, those who do not purchase insurance coverage in some way are penalized via an income tax penalty that will increase in subsequent years.[3,8]

- New models of patient service delivery and payment.
- Increased requirements for demonstrating the value/quality of patient care.
- Increased funding for integrity programs designed to prevent fraud and abuse.[7]

As the implementation of the Affordable Care Act is only partially completed, it is addressed again in this chapter in the section on the future of health-care delivery.

FOR REFLECTION

- Has the implementation of the ACA changed the way in which you access or pay for medical services? If so, in what way? Is this change (or lack of change) a positive or a negative outcome for you?

Current Health-Care Payment Methodology

Assuming patients have health-care insurance, how does the nature of today's health-care environment impact how they are able to receive health-care services? Many patients are facing higher financial responsibility for out-of-pocket deductibles and copayments for office visits, medications, and hospital stays.[3] In addition, insurers often impose limitations on the number of days/visits a patient might be covered for services provided in a designated time frame, sometimes referred to as a "benefit period."[2] Patients may not be eligible for coverage unless the provider contacts the third-party payer prior to delivering the service, a process known as **prior authorization.**[3] In therapy, the number of days authorized is often limited and too few to achieve the goals set in the plan of care; clinicians may need either to contact a payer for reauthorization (sometimes several times throughout an episode of care) or to revise goals to make them more achievable within the given number of visits authorized.[5]

FOR REFLECTION

- Review your medical insurance plan. What coverage do you have for physical therapy? Do you have to pay a copayment for physical therapy? If so, how much is it?

It is impossible for this text to address the specifics of every health insurance plan available to consumers in the United States. However, clinicians in nearly every physical therapy setting will see some patients who have Medicare or Medicaid. In addition, other third-party payers may use Medicare/Medicaid payment regulations as a guide for setting their own policies and criteria. Therefore, PTAs must understand Medicare and Medicaid, how these programs influence the way in which services are provided in their practice settings, and what requirements must be met to receive payment. The following sections review these two programs, highlighting setting-specific criteria and systems that are used for determining and tracking the appropriate charges to be submitted to those payers. Please note that the information is only as current as the date in which it is being written; as regulations often change annually, this information is primarily intended as a guide for the student and should be verified for current accuracy at each setting in which a student performs a clinical experience.

Medicare

Medicare is a federally funded program that is overseen by the **Centers for Medicare & Medicaid Services** (CMS), a division of the U.S. Department of Health and Human Services. With a few rare exceptions, most U.S. citizens are eligible to receive certain Medicare benefits upon turning age 65. Some benefits come without out-of-pocket costs at the time of enrollment, although most people have been paying for Medicare via mandatory payroll deductions throughout their years of employment. Other Medicare benefits are optional and require additional payment. Certain groups of people under age 65 are eligible for Medicare if they demonstrate permanent disability under Social Security guidelines or have end-stage kidney disease.[2]

As mentioned, the first two components of Medicare, Part A and Part B, were created in 1965. Medicare Part C, now also known as Medicare Advantage, was created in 1998. This component of Medicare provides for managed care plans in which Medicare recipients have the option of participating. The extra benefits offered by many of these plans may offset their limitation of having to utilize certain providers within an HMO or PPO.[2] Medicare Part D, which provides elective prescription drug coverage (for a variable monthly cost, depending on the type of coverage desired), was added in 2006.[2] Because physical therapy services billed to Medicare fall under Parts A and B, this text focuses on the specifics of those components.

Medicare A, often referred to as "Hospital Insurance" (and listed as such on one's Medicare card, Fig. 11-1) is the portion of Medicare that comes without payment upon enrollment. It covers most costs incurred while a patient is hospitalized (including physical therapy). In addition, Medicare A may cover portions of a patient's short-term stay in a skilled nursing facility, home care, and hospice services. **Medicare B,** also known as "Medical Insurance," is an elective component that generally covers up to 80 percent of expenses such as physician visits, laboratory testing and imaging, and medically necessary durable medical equipment (DME) ordered by a physician. Types of DME used in physical therapy include items such as walkers, canes, wheelchairs, prosthetics, and orthotics. For 2015, the cost of Medicare B for people with an income of under $85,000 per year is $104.90 per month, with a $147.00 year deductible.[9] In 2013 (the most recent statistics available), approximately 92 percent of Medicare A beneficiaries also opted to purchase Medicare B coverage.[10]

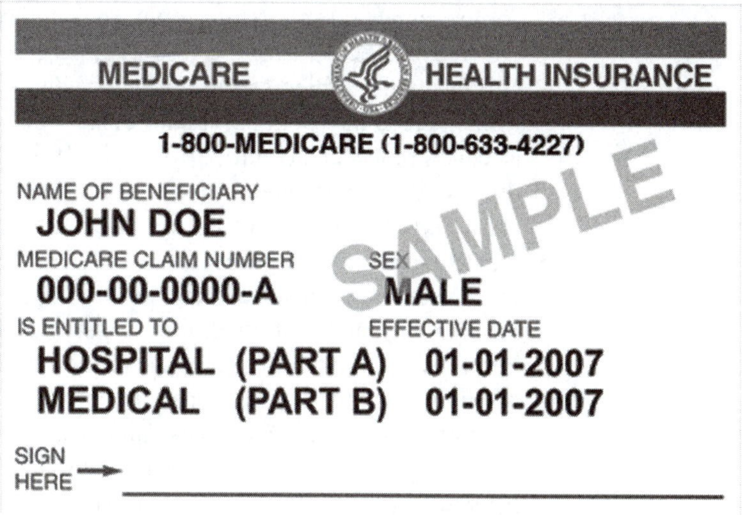

Figure 11-1. Example of a Medicare Card. (Source: Medicare.gov/ medicare-images/Medicare Card.jpg.)

Even if a patient is a Medicare beneficiary, Medicare may or may not cover services delivered during a particular episode of care. The type of Medicare coverage that applies and whether a patient is able to utilize that coverage to pay for PT or other health-care costs depends on a number of factors that include the following:

- The type of facility in which the services are being provided
- Whether the patient needs daily skilled services
- The nature of the functional loss associated with the service
- The overall status of the patient

In acute care, a hospital admission itself qualifies the patient for therapy coverage under Medicare A. However, some patients might stay at a hospital for one or more days "under observation" without actually being admitted; therapy ordered during this period would not be covered under Medicare A, but could be billed under Medicare B (this is addressed in more detail in a subsequent section of this chapter). There are limits to the number of days that Medicare A will provide hospitalization coverage, but given today's short hospital stays, this is rarely an issue for the average patient.

A patient receiving services at home under Medicare A must meet the primary criterion of being considered "homebound." Leaving the home is not forbidden (the patient may leave for medical appointments, religious services, or adult day care), but doing so must require the assistance of another person or excessive effort on the part of the patient to exit the residence. Being unable to drive in and of itself does not qualify a person as being homebound.[9]

In the skilled nursing facility (SNF), Medicare A can provide comprehensive coverage for short-term stays, assuming one or more criteria are met. The essential criterion for this coverage is that the patient has had at least a 3-day hospital admission in the past 30 days. Without this, Medicare A coverage cannot be utilized for that SNF admission. Assuming the hospitalization requirement is met, there must *also* be a need for the patient to have skilled daily nursing or rehabilitation services, as provided by PT, occupational therapist (OT), or a speech-language pathologist.[9] If so, the patient's semiprivate room, meals, medical supplies, and therapy costs will be covered 100 percent for the first 21 days of his stay. If the patient stays longer and still meets the skilled services requirement, his therapy will continue to be paid in full, whereas his room and board costs will be partially covered for up to 100 days, at which point his benefit period ends. If at any time the patient no longer requires daily skilled rehabilitation or nursing services that can be provided appropriately only in an SNF, the patient would no longer be eligible for Medicare A coverage, regardless of at what point he is in his benefit period.[9]

Many permanent residents of an SNF, or those admitted to one without a 3-day hospital stay (as mentioned, this is a situation that is becoming more common as hospitals keep patients under observation without actually admitting them) may still be eligible for therapy coverage under Medicare Part B. This portion of Medicare does not cover room and board, and covers only 80 percent of the therapy charges after the yearly deductible is met. Many patients, however, carry supplemental insurance to cover the portion that Medicare does not. Medicare B would also be the portion of Medicare billed for any services received in an outpatient clinic, or in a hospital when the patient is in an observation unit. Certain outcome measures are required when billing under Medicare B; this is addressed in this chapter's section on coding and billing.

Since 1997, Congress has significantly restricted the total amount of annual coverage for rehabilitation services under Medicare B. This "cap," as it is called, was set for 2015 at $1,940 per year for physical therapy and speech-language pathology services combined, with another $1,940 allotted for occupational therapy services.[11] There are processes for obtaining cap "exceptions" for patients with certain conditions and diagnoses, but in general having the cap in place significantly limits the amount of rehabilitation services that many Medicare B beneficiaries can receive. Since the cap was first introduced, the APTA has fought tirelessly for its elimination. Thanks to the advocacy efforts of thousands of APTA members, there have been several delays in the cap's implementation and many extensions of the time-limited exceptions process, but Congress has yet to rescind the cap completely. At the time of this writing, a Senate vote to do so failed by just two votes, the closest vote yet, but did extend the exceptions process until the end of 2017.[11] APTA leaders remain confident that eventually the cap will be permanently eliminated.

FOR REFLECTION

FOR REFLECTION

- What types of conditions and diagnoses are most likely to exceed the therapy cap most quickly? Why? If this is a challenging question, think about the types of diagnoses and conditions that might require lengthy rehabilitation or services provided by multiple therapies.

Until recently, Medicare held to strict guidelines that allowed rehabilitation providers to bill Medicare for their charges only when there was a reasonable expectation that the patient would demonstrate improvement as a result of receiving those skilled services. Patients whose conditions did not indicate this expectation of improvement could occasionally be seen for a brief period of "specialized maintenance" physical therapy. In these cases, an exercise or mobility program would be established or updated, which would then be carried out by other health-care providers (e.g., nursing staff) or by family members. Beyond this, ongoing PT programs to maintain a patient's condition were not considered to be a skilled service and therefore were not covered. However, as a result of a lawsuit settled in 2013, Medicare published a statement clarifying that skilled services might also be needed to maintain or prevent decline in a patient's status.[12] Medicare's statement indicated that it did not consider this an expansion of its coverage, only a clarification that potential for improvement could not be used by itself as a reason for coverage denial.[12] It is believed that this clarification will result in improved access to rehabilitation for many patients with chronic and/or progressive health conditions.[13]

Medicaid

The **Medicaid** program was created in 1965 via the same legislation that enacted Medicare Parts A and B.[2] However, its focus, funding, and how it is obtained are much different. Medicaid was created to provide medical and long-term care coverage for low-income individuals who were not old enough to qualify for Medicare. Whereas Medicare is a federally funded program, Medicaid is funded by both the federal and state governments, with the federal government covering at least 50 percent of the costs and the state having the responsibility for administering the program.[1] The percentage of funding contributed to the Medicaid program by each state varies depending on a given state's per capita income.[3] States also vary in their eligibility requirements for Medicaid. The federal government mandates that individuals who have already qualified for certain low-income assistance programs or have demonstrated long-term medical needs are automatically eligible for Medicaid in the state in which they live. However, those states may also elect to cover additional groups of individuals and/or may provide differing levels of coverage beyond what is federally required. Because of all these variables from state to state, Medicaid is often referred to as being "fifty different programs."[1]

Because Medicaid is based on income limitations, individuals who have not automatically qualified as described here have to verify their income and assets (or lack thereof). In the case of elderly clients who are facing the high costs of permanent assisted living or skilled nursing placement, qualifying for Medicaid may require them to "spend down" any financial assets they may have to certain low levels before being able to apply. There are some differing requirements in the case of a married couple when only one person requires institutionalized care; for example, the spouse remaining at home is not required to sell their home and can maintain a small income.[3] Children from low-income families are often covered under an expansion of Medicaid now referred to as the Children's Health Insurance Program (CHIP). Most states contract with some type of managed care organization to provide services under Medicaid, believing that it provides recipients greater access to primary care providers at a lower cost.[3]

In recent years, as health-care funding has been debated at the state and national levels, cuts to the Medicaid program's payment for physical therapy services have been common.[14] As part of the ACA, states were initially mandated to increase the coverage they provided via the Medicaid and CHIP programs by raising the minimum income requirements to 138 percent of the poverty level. However, a successful Supreme Court challenge to this policy led to it becoming an optional state decision.[14] If participating, states are required to offer an essential health benefit plan that includes "rehabilitative and habilitative services and devices" through a state health insurance marketplace (also referred to as a health insurance exchange). The incentive for states to participate is a high percentage of federal coverage for those newly eligible (100 percent through 2016) and a lower likelihood of having to absorb health-care costs incurred by people who are uninsured.[14] As of April 2015, 29 states have agreed to expansion, 16 have decided against, and five are undecided.[15]

Payment for physical therapy services provided for people with Medicaid can be made in different ways. If someone has Medicare in addition to Medicaid (a condition known as "dual eligibility"[16]) and the service meets the skilled necessity of Medicare as described in the previous section, then Medicare most often is the primary payer, with Medicaid serving as a secondary payment source that usually covers most of the charges not covered by Medicare.[9] When clients have only Medicaid/CHIP or if the service is not covered under Medicare, the coverage levels will be determined by that state's plan and/or managed care provider, and may include a prior authorization requirement or limitations to the number of visits.[17]

FOR REFLECTION

- What agency regulates Medicaid in your state? Go to that agency's website and find out the percentage that your state contributes to its Medicaid program. Is your state participating in the new expansion program?

Coding and Billing

When PTs and PTAs submit charges for therapies administered to a patient in a given intervention session, they rarely use actual dollar amounts. In most cases, charges for PT services are submitted via the use of certain coding and billing systems. The systems and codes used for billing may be determined by the setting in which the services are provided, the type of insurance (if any) that is paying for the patient's therapy, and the nature of the service provided. In some cases, billing depends on the time spent with the patient. In others, codes are used to bill for each service provided. In addition, coding is also used to classify the patient's medical diagnosis and physical therapy diagnosis. Based on the payment system or setting, specific data must be tracked to ensure payment or to avoid payment penalties.

Diagnostic Coding Systems

Codes that represent the medical diagnosis of a patient are obtained from the **International Classification of Diseases (ICD),** a compilation put together by the

World Health Organization. Originally the ICD was designed to track global causes of mortality, but a clinical modification (CM) version was subsequently created for use in tracking diagnoses in inpatient and outpatient care, and was later updated to include inpatient procedural codes. These codes are also used to categorize a patient's physical therapy diagnosis, which often differs from the medical diagnosis. The previous version, ICD-9-CM, containing just over 14,000 diagnosis codes and 3,800 procedure codes, was replaced by a much more complex version, ICD-10-CM, on October 1, 2015. The ICD-10-CM is much more detailed, with nearly 70,000 diagnoses and almost 72,000 procedures, using a more extensive identifying system (see Fig. 11-2).[18]

FOR REFLECTION

- Why does a patient's diagnosis need to be coded so specifically? Identify at least one purpose for which a specific code might be used.

Physical Therapy Procedural Coding Systems

Every activity performed with patients in physical therapy also has a procedural code connected to it. Some are very specific, whereas others are more broad. The system now used in physical therapy is called **Current Procedural Terminology (CPT)** coding. It was developed by the American Medical Association (AMA) and is used not only by medicine and physical therapy, but also by many other health professions. Since the inception of CPT coding in the mid-1990s, the APTA has provided feedback and worked closely with members of the AMA to better refine the codes used by physical therapists (Fig 11-2).[19]

FOR REFLECTION

- Two codes commonly used in physical therapy are 97110 and 97530 (see Fig. 11-2). What are the differences between those two codes? Give an example of an intervention that would fall into each category.

Once a CPT code is established, the charge associated with it must be determined. Not all components of intervention are created equally; some have a greater charge associated with them than do others. The dollar amount associated with each code is a measure of its "relative value" compared with other interventions. The **Resource-Based Relative Value Scale** (RBRVS) is the most commonly used method for determining what these fees should be. The RBRVS assigns a value to each CPT code, taking into consideration the work involved to perform a given component—not just the physical skill, but also the required knowledge, the amount of decision-making, and potential risk—then figuring in the clinic expense, the malpractice costs, and the geographic region in which the care is being provided.[2] When used by Medicare, the RBRVS amounts are then multiplied by a conversion factor determined annually by Congress and CMS. The rates are then published as the **Physician Fee Schedule** (PFS).[2] All health professions that use CPT codes use the PFS to determine

97110	Therapeutic exercises to develop strength and endurance, range of motion, and flexibility (15 minutes)
97140	Manual therapy techniques (e.g., connective tissue massage, joint mobilization and manipulation, and manual traction) (15 minutes)
97010	Hot or cold pack application
97014	Electrical stimulation (unattended)
97112	Neuromuscular re-education of movement, balance, coordination, kinesthetic sense, posture, and/or proprioception for sitting and/or standing activities (15 minutes)
97001	Physical therapy evaluation
97530	Dynamic activities to improve functional performance, direct (one-on-one) with the patient (15 minutes)
97035	Ultrasound (15 minutes)
97002	Physical therapy re-evaluation
97032	Electrical stimulation (manual) (15 minutes)
97116	Gait training (includes stair climbing) (15 minutes)
97012	Mechanical traction
97113	Aquatic therapy with therapeutic exercises (15 minutes)

Figure 11-2. CPT Codes Commonly Used in Physical Therapy. (Copyright American Medical Association.)

their anticipated payment.[2,19] However, not all codes can be used by all providers, and some payers will not cover certain codes when used in physical therapy.[19]

CPT codes generally are updated on a yearly basis; new codes are added, others eliminated, and interpretations of situations in which certain ones should be used may be changed. In addition, CMS and congressional edicts may affect coding criteria, change the values of those factors that determine the fee schedule, or create new formulas for determining proper payment. It is extremely important to keep up to date with any changes to assure full payment for services performed.

Additional Payment Systems for Health-Care Services

Using codes as the primary way to request payment is part of the traditional **fee for service** model of reimbursement in which a provider performs a service first and then requests payment after the fact.[2] This method, although probably the one that is the most clear concerning the actual services provided, potentially could encourage providers to perform and charge for excessive services that may not have actually been needed.[2,20] Other methods of payment include "per diem" payment (lump sum payment per day of service or intervention session, regardless of what was provided), lump sum payments per episode of care to individual providers, or lump sum monthly payments to a provider group or setting that covers multiple disciplines, regardless of the number of patients seen or the services provided. This last method of payment is known as capitation. A form of capitation is seen in hospitals, where Medicare payments are made based on **diagnosis-related groups** (DRGs) into which patients are categorized, regardless of the severity of illness, length of stay, or services provided.[1,20]

Setting-Specific Payment Determination Tools and Outcome Measurement Requirements

Depending on the payer source, codes may not necessarily be the only deciding factor in what PT departments are paid. There are other tools that clinicians must use to determine the appropriate amounts billed to Medicare or other providers, based on the different payment systems that are in place for that payer in that setting. DRGs are one example of a **prospective payment system** (PPS), in which providers are aware of the predetermined payment they will be receiving prior to delivering care.[2,3] Medicare has been using this system for hospital inpatient services since 1983, and in 2000, as a result of the Balanced Budget Act of 1997, added two additional prospective payment systems for Medicare A patients in the SNF and home care settings. Both of these require different comprehensive assessment tools to be completed by multiple providers at certain times during a patient's episode of care. In home care, billing under Medicare requires the use of a tool called the **Outcomes and Assessment Information Set** (OASIS) to collect data on a given patient's functional status. These data then determine which one of 153 lump sum rates will be paid for the services during each 60-day benefit period.[2]

In the SNF, a different PPS is used. In this setting, the complexity of the patient's medical status places him or her into one of 66 **Resource Utilization Groups** (RUGs) that reflect the total potential makeup of a facility's population, also known as its **case mix.**[21] Multiple providers within the SNF assess each patient's abilities, based on parameters set for their discipline, using a document called the **Minimum Data Set** (MDS). Part of what determines the patient's case mix index is the number of minutes of daily skilled therapy services that he needs. This number is predicted at the beginning of the patient's stay, but if the predicted number of therapy minutes cannot actually be provided and/or is not documented on the MDS during designated periods, the patient will not meet the expected RUG level, and the payment to the facility will be less than anticipated. PPS was designed as an improvement on excessive fee-for-service claims, in that payment for therapy services is built into the RUG level rather than being an additional charge. However, linking increased payment to additional therapy minutes has potentially encouraged overprovision of services, that is, every patient may be classified as needing the minutes required for the highest levels of reimbursement. It also presents clinicians with ethical challenges when being encouraged to maximize the billable minutes of therapy provided at times when that might be considered contraindicated or inappropriate.[22] Aware of the need for reform in this area, Congress recently enacted legislation, the Improving Medicare Post-Acute Care Transformation (IMPACT) Act of 2014, aimed to address these concerns. This legislation is addressed later in this chapter.

Medicare A is not alone in having special requirements for payment. In 2012, new federal legislation was enacted that began requiring rehabilitation providers billing for services under Medicare B to begin a process known as functional limitations reporting, in hopes of collecting data that will help influence future health-care legislation and practices.[23] Providers submit data to Medicare via the use of specific nonbillable **G-codes,** based on ICF categories of disability (see Chapter 2). There are currently 14 G-code categories (six of which are primarily used by PT or OT), with three codes within each of those categories. Clinicians must code the category that is most relevant to that patient situation, the point in the episode of care that the limitation is being assessed (initially, at specifically designated times during the episode of care, and at discharge) and the severity of the patient's limitation at that point.[24] Failure to do so will result in denial of the patient's Medicare claim.[23]

In addition to G-codes, private practice providers billing under Medicare Part B must also report on certain patient outcome measures by using the **Physician Quality Reporting System** (PQRS). When first established in 2007, this was an elective, incentive-based system (providers received a financial benefit for participating) but, via the adoption of the ACA, it was changed to a system that is penalty based (as of 2015, providers who haven't been participating will face reductions in what Medicare pays them for services provided).[25] The purpose of having clinicians report specific data is to create a higher level of care and a higher level of accountability. Doing so is part of the overall trend of payment systems moving toward paying for the value of the services provided (as measured by outcomes) rather than arbitrarily paying for any services provided.[25,26] The details of which outcomes need to be assessed and the penalties assessed for not doing so have changed annually. As of 2015, private practice clinics generally need to report on nine of 15 different measures (including at least one that is measured by multiple disciplines to allow for comparisons) on at least 50 percent of their patients seen under Medicare B.[25]

Tracking and submitting patient outcomes data, in addition to the usual documentation and billing, can be confusing and is time consuming. Clinicians can submit these data with each claim submitted for payment, but as submission requirements have become more complicated, more clinicians are moving toward utilizing a qualified registry system to collate and submit the data.[9,25] The APTA has recently begun piloting the use of its own physical therapy outcomes registry. Using a PT-specific registry will not only assist clinicians in submitting their data, but will also contribute to health-care reform by promoting higher levels of practice and research through the collection of outcomes that demonstrate physical therapy's effectiveness.[27]

FOR REFLECTION

FOR REFLECTION
_____

- What physical therapy outcomes do you think are most important to measure? Go to CMS's or the APTA's website to find the current list of outcome measures used. Are the ones you identified on the list?

The Future of Health-Care Policy and Payment Systems

The goals of the "triple aim" continue to be reflected in the elements of the ACA and the increasing regulations of Medicare and other third-party payers. The IMPACT Act mandated the expansion of reporting requirements to include all post-acute care settings, such as SNFs, home care, and inpatient rehabilitation facilities, using standardized measures that can be assessed across the continuum of care.[28] Therefore, most health-care providers and settings are now required to use or are moving toward some type of quality reporting system. In these systems, payment is tied to achieving successful outcomes, and providers and/or facilities may be penalized when additional care or readmission to a facility is required.[11] These regulations expect a new level of provider collaboration. New integrated care models such as **accountable care organizations** (ACOs), medical homes, and coordinated health networks are becoming much more common,[29] as are models in which organizations receive one "bundled" payment for services provided by multiple providers.[30] These new frameworks require increased teamwork among providers to minimize duplication of services and to ensure that the most appropriate providers work with a given patient to provide the best value and obtain the best outcomes.[30] The growing evidence that early physical therapy for musculoskeletal injuries is more cost effective[31,32] is positioning the profession to be a key player in the provision of value-based services.[33]

Another payment-related trend is the growth of cash-based physical therapy practices.[20] In this setup, providers do not work with Medicare or other third-party payers, and all services are delivered on a fee-for-service basis that the patient pays out of pocket. This allows for a more consistent cash flow because clinics do not have to submit claims and then wait for payment from a third-party payer. Clients who have physical therapy benefits under their insurance plan may incur higher costs by seeing a cash-only provider than they would with a provider contracted through their payer. However, many of the individuals receiving services in these types of payment models have frequently exhausted their benefits or no longer qualify for services under their policy guidelines.[20]

A more broad concern for the future of health care is the ease and availability of access to the system. There is currently a shortage of traditional primary care providers (physicians, nurse practitioners, and physician assistants), especially in underserved areas, and this trend is expected to worsen in coming years.[1,2] The current entry-level education for Doctors of Physical Therapy in screening and systems review, along with the evidence that physical therapists are effective in a direct access model, may lead to the profession as a whole seeking recognition as a primary care provider that could ease those shortages.[33]

The APTA's Advocacy Efforts Related to Health-Care Policy and Payment

One of the major areas of focus for APTA staff and members is to advocate for legislative and regulatory changes in health-care payment and policy that will benefit physical therapy patients and providers. Every two years, at the start of a new congressional session, the APTA's Public Policy and Advocacy Committee (PPAC) issues its "Public Policy Priorities," those issues that are most pressing and require the most attention so that the APTA may achieve the goals of its mission and strategic plan.[34] These and other issues may be addressed in meetings with payers, in formal communication with regulatory agencies (often in response to proposed or enacted rules that impact physical therapy service access or delivery), or by visiting members of Congress to solicit their support for certain health-care legislation. The advocacy efforts are not just at the federal level, however. The APTA also has staff that helps chapters respond to legislative or regulatory issues that arise in their state. For individual members, the APTA provides many resources to help with questions concerning payment, coding and billing, payment models, and health-care reform on their website. The site's **Legislative Action Center** allows members to send personalized letters to their state or federal legislators on a variety of issues with just a couple of clicks.[35] Other ways in which PTs and PTAs can support the APTA's work in this area are addressed in the final section of this chapter.

The APTA is taking a proactive stance on fraud, abuse, and waste in the health-care system. Our historical models of payment (and some of our current ones) have unfortunately perpetuated the opportunity for illegal, unethical, and unprofessional behaviors, and the profession of physical therapy is not exempt from these kinds of problems. As defined in Chapter 10, fraud related to payment generally refers to *deliberate* falsification of billing records, whereas abuse describes an *unintentional* error, such as unknowingly using the wrong billing code.[36,37] In order to have a credible voice in reform and advocacy efforts, the APTA has taken a proactive stance in dealing with issues related to fraud and abuse via the implementation of an **Integrity in Practice campaign** to educate clinicians more thoroughly on the problems related to fraud and abuse.[38] Among the tools being used to do so is the document "Primer on Fraud and Abuse," located on the APTA Center for Integrity in Practice website,[38] and an online continuing education course available for free to members and nonmembers (including students) via the APTA's Learning Center. "Navigating the Regulatory Environment: Ensuring Compliance While Promoting Professional Integrity" uses cases based on real-life situations to educate participants about the ways in which fraud and abuse have occurred in physical therapy, and provides best-practice examples of how to ensure compliance with rules and regulations.[39]

In addition to educating clinicians on fraud and abuse, the Integrity in Practice campaign also seeks to promote the provision of value-based care.[38] Another way that the APTA is contributing to this goal is through the development of a new model for physical therapy coding and billing. Currently called the **Physical Therapy Classification and Payment System** (PTCPS), it seeks to overhaul the present CPT codes used to bill for physical therapy services. Instead of codes that are based on physical therapy tasks and interventions, clinicians will bill using codes that reflect the criticality of the patient receiving the service and the complexity of the skill provided, without being specific to a given procedure. Members of the APTA are working closely with the AMA (as the "owners" of the CPT coding system) on this new system. The current focus of this work is on new evaluation and re-evaluation codes. These are expected to be released by the AMA in the fall of 2016 for use beginning in 2017.[40]

Assisting in APTA Advocacy Efforts

Although the APTA has a strong, well-respected staff constantly advocating for patients and the profession, they cannot do this work alone. Membership in the APTA is one simple way of providing support. Each member adds to the collective size of our organization—and an organization with a larger total membership often garners more attention and potentially has greater clout during interactions with government officials and legislators. Becoming a member also provides the APTA with greater financial resources to help fund its public policy work. A different way of contributing to the financial resources needed to fight legislative battles is to support the Physical Therapy Political Action Committee (PT-PAC), which raises funds that are used strategically to gain access to and support from legislators.[41] PTs, PTAs, and students are also encouraged to become part of the grassroots network to create a critical mass of voices reaching out to government officials. The APTA Legislative Action Center is a quick, efficient way of reaching your legislators; there is also a link on the APTA's advocacy page that can be used by patients to contact their legislators on key issues. If one is more comfortable advocating in person, many states have designated "Legislative Days" in which coordinated groups of members visit legislators at their state capitol. Similar mass advocacy events are also organized by the APTA twice a year at the national level.

Other ways to support the APTA's efforts include joining the **PTeam** to receive regular updates on advocacy issues and notice of important times to contact your legislators regarding impending legislative votes. PTeam members who want a higher level of involvement may choose to become a **Key Contact,** a position in which one takes responsibility for developing a relationship with one's legislators and coordinating advocacy efforts with other members of the physical therapy community in that legislative district. Experienced members who want a greater role in directing their chapter's or section's legislative efforts can become a State or Federal Legislative Affairs Liaison, serving as the official point of contact between the APTA and that component, or can consider being appointed to the PPAC.[35]

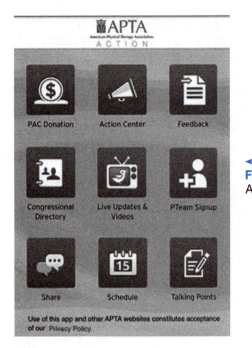

Figure 11-3. Features of the APTA Advocacy App for iPhone and Android.

Access to these opportunities for being involved and taking action is available through the APTA's online advocacy page, but they can also be accessed with an APTA Advocacy app that is available to members and nonmembers (see Fig. 11-3).

S U M M A R Y

Paying for health care has become much more complicated and much more expensive over the past century. As managed care has become more prevalent, providers are struggling with decreased payments for and increased restrictions on the services they are allowed to provide. The ramifications of the Affordable Care Act are yet to be fully realized, but have already led to philosophical and regulatory changes in the health-care environment, including an increased emphasis on providing value and demonstrating accountability via outcomes and a push for greater integration of health-care delivery among providers. Despite the frequency in which providers see patients covered under Medicare, the increased regulation and the variation in coverage and reporting requirements from setting to setting make keeping up with all of the appropriate rules very challenging. Staying connected with the APTA is a primary way to ensure that one has the most up-to-date information. The APTA has many ways in which it attempts to improve access for patients and maximize payment for clinicians via advocacy at the state and national levels, but needs the grassroots support of the membership for it to be more effective in its lobbying efforts.

REFERENCES

1. Sultz HA, Young KM. *Health Care, USA: Understanding Its Organization and Delivery.* 8th ed. Sudbury, MA: Jones & Bartlett; 2014.

2. Shi L, Singh DA. *Essentials of the US Health Care System.* Sudbury, MA: Jones & Bartlett; 2010.

3. Feldstein PJ. *Health Policy Issues: An Economic Perspective on Health Reform.* 5th ed. Chicago, IL: Health Administration Press; 2011.

4. Bodenheimer T, Grumbach K. *Understanding Health Policy: A Clinical Approach.* 6th ed. New York, NY: McGraw-Hill; 2012:231.

5. Sandstrom R, Lohman H, Bramble J. *Health Services Policy and Systems for Therapists.* Upper Saddle River, NJ: Prentice Hall; 2003:292.

6. Berwick D, Nolan T, Whittington J. The triple aim: care, health, and cost. *Health Aff.* 27:759-769.

7. American Physical Therapy Association. Health care reform. http://www.apta.org/HealthCareReform/. Updated 2013. Accessed April 21, 2015.

8. Centers for Medicare & Medicaid Services. Fees and exemptions overview. HealthCare.gov Web site. https://www.healthcare.gov/fees-exemptions/. Updated 2015. Accessed April 30, 2015.

9. Centers for Medicare & Medicaid Services. Medicare.gov: The official US government site for Medicare. http://www.medicare.gov/what-medicare-covers/index.html. Accessed April 20, 2015.

10. National Committee to Preserve Social Security and Medicare. Fast facts about Medicare. http://www.ncpssm.org/Medicare/MedicareFastFacts. Updated 2015. Accessed April 21, 2015.

11. American Physical Therapy Association. Medicare payment and reimbursement. http://www.apta.org/Medicare/. Updated 2015. Accessed April 21, 2015.

12. Centers for Medicare & Medicaid Services. Therapy services: *Jimmo v. Sebelius* settlement agreement—program manual clarifications (fact sheet). http://www.cms.gov/Medicare/Billing/TherapyServices/index.html. Updated 2015. Accessed April 21, 2015.

13. Rockar PA Jr. Statement by APTA president on settlement of Medicare "improvement standard" class action lawsuit. American Physical Therapy Association Web site. http://www.apta.org/Media/Releases/Legislative/2013/2/8/. Updated 2013. Accessed April 21, 2015.

14. American Physical Therapy Association. Medicaid. APTA.org Web site. http://www.apta.org/Payment/Medicaid/. Updated 2014. Accessed April 22, 2015.

15. Kaiser Family Foundation. Status of state action on the Medicaid expansion decision. Henry J. Kaiser Family Foundation Web site. http://kff.org/health-reform/state-indicator/state-activity-around-expanding-medicaid-under-the-affordable-care-act/. Updated 2015. Accessed April 27, 2015.

16. Centers for Medicare & Medicaid Services. Seniors & Medicare and Medicaid enrollees. Medicaid.gov Web site. http://medicaid.gov/medicaid-chip-program-information/by-population/medicare-medicaid-enrollees-dual-eligibles/seniors-and-medicare-and-medicaid-enrollees.html. Updated 2015. Accessed April 27, 2015.

17. National Council on Disability. Medicare managed care for people with disabilities: policy and implementation considerations for state and federal policymakers. 2013.

18. Centers for Disease Control and Prevention. International classification of diseases, tenth revision, clinical modification (ICD-10-CM). CDC.gov Web site. http://www.cdc.gov/nchs/icd/icd10cm.htm. Updated 2015. Accessed April 30, 2015.

19. American Physical Therapy Association. Coding and billing. APTA.org Web site. http://www.apta.org/Payment/CodingBilling/. Updated 2015. Accessed April 22, 2015.

20. American Physical Therapy Association. Payment methodologies: advantages vs. disadvantages for practice. APTA.org Web site. http://www.apta.org/Payment/ PrivateInsurance/PaymentMethodologies/. Updated 2014. Accessed April 22, 2015.

21. Centers for Medicare & Medicaid Services. Skilled nursing facility PPS. CMS. gov Web site. http://www.cms.gov/Medicare/Medicare-Fee-for-Service-Payment/ SNFPPS/index.html. Updated 2013. Accessed April 22, 2015.

22. Hayhurst C. Fighting fraud and abuse in physical therapy. *PT in Motion*. 2012;(6).

23. American Physical Therapy Association. Functional limitation reporting under Medicare. APTA.org Web site. http://www.apta.org/Payment/Medicare/ CodingBilling/FunctionalLimitation/. Updated 2015. Accessed April 22, 2015.

24. Centers for Medicare & Medicaid Services. Functional reporting. CMS.gov Web site. http://www.cms.gov/Medicare/Billing/TherapyServices/Functional-Reporting .html. Updated 2014. Accessed April 22, 2015.

25. Smith HL. Update on the physician quality reporting system. *PT in Motion*. 2015;7(3):8-9, 12.

26. American Physical Therapy Association. Medicare physician quality reporting system (PQRS). APTA.org Web site. http://www.apta.org/PQRS/. Updated 2015. Accessed April 27, 2015.

27. American Physical Therapy Association. Physical therapy outcomes registry. http://www.ptoutcomes.com/Home.aspx. Updated 2015. Accessed April 23, 2015.

28. Centers for Medicare & Medicaid Services. IMPACT Act of 2014 & cross setting measures. CMS.gov Web site. http://cms.gov/Medicare/Quality-Initiatives-Patient -Assessment-Instruments/Post-Acute-Care-Quality-Initiatives/IMPACT-Act-of -2014-and-Cross-Setting-Measures.html. Updated 2015. Accessed May 2, 2015.

29. Plymale J. Stop struggling to find your place in new integrated care delivery models. *PPS Impact*. May 2015.

30. Worth R. Surviving and thriving: how to stay successful in the new world of health care. *PPS Impact*. May 2015.

31. Pendergast J, Kliethermes SA, Freburger JK, Duffy PA. A comparison of health care use for physician-referred and self-referred episodes of outpatient physical therapy. *Health Serv Res*. 2012;47(2):633-654.

32. Chou R, Rothschild B. Review: evidence for the effectiveness of nonsurgical interventions for low back pain and radiculopathy is limited. *ACP J Club*. 2009;151(4):7-7.

33. Jewell DV, Moore JD, Goldstein MS. Delivering the physical therapy value proposition: a call to action. *Phys Ther*. 2013;93(1):104-114.
34. American Physical Therapy Association. APTA's 2015-2016 public policy priorities. http://www.apta.org/FederalIssues/PublicPolicyPriorities/. Updated 2015. Accessed April 30, 2015.
35. American Physical Therapy Association. Advocacy. APTA.org Web site. http://www.apta.org/Advocacy/. Updated 2014. Accessed April 30, 2015.
36. Nicholson S. *The Physical Therapist's Business Practice and Legal Guide*. Sudbury, MA: Jones & Bartlett; 2008:399.
37. Nosse LJ, Friberg DG, Kovacek PR. *Managerial and Supervisory Principles for Physical Therapists*. 2nd ed. Baltimore, MD: Lippincott Williams & Wilkins; 2005.
38. American Physical Therapy Association. APTA Center for Integrity in Practice. APTA.org Web site. http://integrity.apta.org/home.aspx. Updated 2015. Accessed April 27, 2015.
39. American Physical Therapy Association. Navigating the regulatory environment: ensuring compliance while promoting professional integrity. APTA.org Web site. http://www.apta.org/Courses/Online/NavigatingCompliance/. Updated 2014. Accessed April 27, 2015.
40. American Physical Therapy Association. Statement by APTA president on 2016 Progress Toward Payment Reform. APTA.org Web site. http://www.apta.org/Media/Releases/Association/2016/5/24/. Updated 2016. Accessed August 1, 2016.
41. Physical Therapy Political Action Committee. About PT-PAC. PTPAC.org Web site. http://www.ptpac.org/about_ptpac. Updated 2015. Accessed April 30, 2015.

Name _____

REVIEW

1. List the three components of the "triple aim."

_____

_____

_____

2. For each of the following acronyms, provide the term that is being abbreviated.

    a. PQRS   _____

    b. MDS   _____

    c. CPT   _____

    d. CMS   _____

    e. PT-PAC   _____

    f. OASIS   _____

    g. RBRVS   _____

    h. PPS   _____

    i. ICD   _____

    j. ACO   _____

3. Match each term in question 2 with its correct definition.

_____ Multidisciplinary document used in the SNF setting to collect patient information, including the number of minutes each patient receives PT.

_____ Agency within the U.S. Department of Health and Human Services that regulates government insurance programs

_____ World Health Organization codes used to categorize medical and PT diagnoses

_____ New care model in which providers share responsibility for providing services and achieving outcomes

(questions continue on page 220)

_____ Requires private practice clinicians providing services under Medicare B to report on specific outcome measures or face payment reductions

_____ Billing codes developed by the American Medical Association; used by a PT to indicate what services were provided

_____ Allows providers to know the payment that will be received for a service, prior to it being delivered

_____ Division of the APTA that uses donated funds to support its public policy and advocacy efforts

_____ Used to determine the fee that should be associated with a given procedure, by taking into consideration the skill, knowledge, decision-making, and risk involved

_____ Tool used in the home health setting to collect data on a patient's functional status

Application

Linda is a 72-year-old who lives with her spouse in a multilevel town house with three steps to climb to enter it. She has Medicare Parts A and B, and also has a Medicare supplement. Linda has severe chronic left knee pain as a result of osteoarthritis, and chooses to have a total knee replacement for pain relief. She is admitted to the hospital for surgery and postsurgical PT and OT. After 3 days, Linda is transferred to a transitional care unit (TCU) of a skilled nursing facility (SNF) for further rehabilitation. She remains there for 10 days, and then is discharged to her home. After returning home, she receives PT for 3 more weeks and is discharged from PT after having met her goals of independent community ambulation with the use of a single-end care, independent stair climbing, independent transfers including in/out of the bathtub, and left knee range of motion of 0 degrees to 135 degrees.

Based on this information, answer the following questions:

1. To which form of Medicare were Linda's hospitalization charges billed?

_____

2. In the hospital, what percentage of her room/therapy charges were most likely covered?

_____

3. To which form of Medicare were Linda's TCU charges billed?

_____

4. In the TCU, what percentage of Linda's room/therapy charges were most likely covered?

_____

5. If Linda had stayed in the hospital for only 2 days, how would that have changed

the billing for her room and therapy charges in the TCU? _____

_____

_____

6. At the time of discharge from the TCU, Linda is able to go up and down a flight of stairs with contact guard assistance, and needs occasional assistance to lift her left lower extremity when getting in and out of the car. Based on this status and Linda's desire to minimize her out-of-pocket costs, would Linda's PT be more likely to recommend home care or an outpatient clinic for continued PT? Explain the rationale for your response. How would insurance cover her PT in that setting?

_____

_____

_____

_____

_____

_____

12

Leadership Development for Physical Therapist Assistants

CHAPTER OBJECTIVES

After reading this chapter, the reader will be able to:

- Discuss traditional and nontraditional views of leadership.
- Discuss current health-care leadership trends.
- List traits that are currently used to exemplify leadership.
- Recognize why physical therapist assistants (PTAs) need to develop or enhance their leadership skills.
- Recognize leadership traits in himself and others.
- Identify ways in which leadership skills can be developed.
- Plan a course of action for his own leadership development.

KEY TERMS AND CONCEPTS

- Leadership versus management
- Shared responsibility
- Leadership traits
- Functional leadership
- Entry-level PTA traits
- Self-reflection
- "Professional Behaviors for the 21st Century"
- Leadership, Administration, Management, and Professionalism (LAMP) certificate program

D *aniel recently enrolled in a PTA program at his local community college. This week, in his Introduction to Physical Therapy class, the scheduled topic is leadership development. Daniel assumes this is going to be about how physical therapists (PTs) develop as leaders or how he and his classmates might develop leadership skills by going on for further education after graduating from the PTA program. The instructor asks the class, "How many of you think that you are going to be a leader in your first job?" Like most of his classmates, Daniel does*

(vignette continues on page 224)

not raise his hand. However, he is taken aback when his instructor tells them that even in their first job they will all need to demonstrate leadership abilities to be successful as a PTA. Daniel asks his instructor, "Why does a PTA need to be a leader? The PT is always the one in charge, not the PTA."

QUESTIONS TO CONSIDER

What does it mean to be a leader? What are the expectations for leadership in today's clinical environment? How is this demonstrated in the work of the PTA? Are leadership traits needed by PTs different from those needed by PTAs? Can leadership be taught?

The opening scenario is a typical one. Most students entering a PTA program do not seem to think of themselves as leaders or at least do not think that leadership traits are an essential component of being an effective PTA. After all, they will argue, doesn't a PTA have to work under the "direction and supervision" of a PT?[1] As this mantra is repeated over and over by faculty throughout students' time in their educational programs, especially early on, it is not surprising that many students do not recognize that an entry-level PTA needs to develop the same leadership skills as does an entry-level PT.[2] Before discussing why these traits are so important, it may be helpful to define what leadership is and what it is not.

Leadership Versus Management

Many people tend to equate leadership with management. The role of a manager has been defined as someone who directs the activities of others.[3] In terms of leadership, people with management positions within an organization or a department have traditionally been thought of as leaders, whereas those being directed by them have been considered followers, expected to perform as directed. Although someone in a traditional management role can certainly exhibit leadership traits, many now consider management and leadership as two separate roles with overlapping but different skill sets. A manager has been understood to be someone who maintains consistency and order in an organization, whereas a leader is someone who motivates, establishes direction, and creates change.[2,4,5] Along these lines, leadership now is defined less often by a formal title that puts someone "in charge" of people and decision-making and more often as a skill set that anyone can develop, no matter what his position may be.[4]

More and more, successful businesses are recognizing that leadership needs to be a **shared responsibility** among multiple people within an organization.[3,6–11] In a shared leadership model, persons in traditional leadership positions delegate decision-making responsibilities to other individuals or groups of individuals within the organization, many of whom are in positions not traditionally associated with leadership. Individuals are expected to perform without constant oversight or delegation. Committees within organizations often have representation from multiple levels of responsibility, and these groups are often empowered to make decisions for the organization as a whole, out of the need to respond rapidly to change.[4,12–14]

In health care, similar trends are being seen out of this same necessity. The term "chaos" has been used in the past to describe the state of health care.[13-15] Care providers, patients, and health-care executives are all generally unsatisfied with the current state of health care.[6,12,16,17] Scientific and technological advances have led to medical care that is increasingly more effective but also more complex and expensive.[6,13,16] The range of health needs is diverse. People are living longer and are choosing to receive medical care in a variety of settings. Confusing payment systems that regulate service delivery are fluid and often poorly defined. Change has become a constant. Because of all this, it has become impractical and ineffective for just one or a few individuals to have the only responsibility for decision-making, innovation, or ensuring the quality of care. As traditional leaders function at capacity, their need to share responsibility is creating nontraditional leadership demands from those at all levels of the health-care organization.[8,9,12,18,19]

Leadership Traits

What makes an effective leader? A search of any media retailer's inventory will yield many hits related to the topic of leadership. Although these resources address leadership from multiple approaches, they identify similar traits as essential for demonstration of successful leadership.[8] The work of Kouzes and Posner is a frequently cited example.[7,8,20] These researchers identify essential practices of leadership that include being able to envision change and then communicating that vision in a way that inspires others to share in it. Other practices they recognize as essential include the following:

- Modeling desired behaviors with words and actions
- Encouraging others
- Being comfortable in challenging existing processes
- Empowering others to take action[7]

Today's leaders facilitate the development of leadership strength in others by acknowledging that they don't have all the answers and by recruiting others to share in the decision-making and effectiveness of the organization.[7,8,19]

In health care, the same need exists for new leadership strengths, and the same traits are being demanded of those working in it. Behaviors cited in current literature as essential for health-care leaders include being able to handle stress and change, having an ability to recognize when change does and doesn't need to happen, possessing highly developed senses of self-discipline and initiative, and having an inner drive to constantly grow and learn.[10,21] Dye and Garman, in writing about essential skills needed by health-care executives, cite behaviors that mirror those noted by Kouzes and Posner. In addition, they state that today's health-care leader must have a strong self-concept. This includes possessing "emotional intelligence," which they define as "understanding and working with other people's emotions while understanding and managing your own personal responses."[22] Dye and Garman also stress the need for strong interpersonal and communication skills, which include using active listening strategies (see Chapter 6) and displaying sensitivity to others when giving them constructive feedback.[22] In promoting shared decision-making and leadership development, many of today's health-care leaders encourage the use of **functional leadership,** rotating people in and out of leadership roles as needed for different tasks and projects based on their interests, unique skill sets, and knowledge bases.[23]

FOR REFLECTION

■ Do you agree that the traits identified above represent leadership traits? Do you possess any of these traits right now?

Leadership Needs in Physical Therapy

Are the traits identified in the previous section needed in the physical therapy profession? Research supports that they are being sought after in PT graduates. In a study of New York clinicians who were asked about hiring criteria for entry-level PTs, the most important abilities looked for included strong communication skills (oral and written), professionalism, and strong time-management skills.[24] But what about the requirements for PTAs? Very little published research has been conducted on the PTA's need to demonstrate leadership traits as a formally identified skill set. However, in a study performed by this author,[25] clinical instructors (CIs) were asked to identify the most important **entry-level PTA traits.** Among the choices offered within the survey, those recognized most frequently as "most important" were the following:

- Being able to recognize changes in the patient's status
- Appearing confident in one's own abilities
- Being able to manage time independently during patient interventions
- Being able to independently decide how to progress or modify delivery of a patient's intervention within the plan of care
- Being able to respond to variations in the daily schedule without demonstrating stress

Respondents to this survey were also asked to write in any behavioral traits not specifically listed within the survey that they felt were "most important." The top traits the CIs added to this list included the following:

- Having strong oral and written communication skills
- Demonstrating a strong interest in learning and an ability to teach others

- Having a positive personality
- Being competent and knowledgeable
- Demonstrating high levels of responsibility

Although all of the traits included in this survey were not explicitly labeled "leadership" traits (to avoid biasing any respondents who had a preconceived idea of what "leadership" should entail), they certainly correlate with those identified as desired traits in entry-level PTs and, more important, correlate with what the literature defines as "leadership."[8,14,21,22,25,26]

Can leadership be taught? Can a PTA learn how to be a leader? In years past, it was believed that leaders were "born" and that leadership was not a trait that could develop. However, that train of thought appears to be less prevalent now.[3,4,8] The abundance of resources on the subject would tend to support the notion that leadership skills can be developed just like any other skill set. Many educational institutions now offer a master's or doctorate degree in leadership or a related area. However, just as one does not need a high-level position or title to need leadership skills in the workplace, one does not have to obtain a high-level degree to develop skills in this area. Conversely, one should not assume that someone who has a more advanced degree has better developed leadership skills.

FOR REFLECTION
FOR REFLECTION

■ Do you think that a person can learn to be a leader? Why or why not?

Recognizing PTA Leadership Demands

Future (or current) PTAs who may still be questioning the need for leadership on their part may want to consider leadership expectations from the patient's perspective. In any encounter that occurs between the patient and the PTA, who will the patient expect to direct the course of the treatment session? Who will make decisions about how to advance or modify that plan, depending on what happens during the course of intervention delivery? The patient's input is always essential and should be sought out, but the decision-making responsibilities in any given treatment session are always part of the PTA's role even if some of those decisions may include obtaining the input of the supervising PT. When a PTA is the primary provider of physical therapy services within a given intervention session, he is expected to be an effective communicator, demonstrating confidence and needing minimal direction while delivering timely and effective interventions. The PTA also is expected to take an active role in departmental efficiency and effectiveness, balancing the challenges of maximizing patient satisfaction, being fiscally responsible, and operating in an ethical and legal manner at all times. This *is* leadership as required in the current health-care environment, and PTAs should feel an obligation to develop these traits.[27]

PTAs should also recognize that their previous life experiences may have already enabled them to develop skills that haven't traditionally been associated with leadership but that are now recognized as part of this skill set. The student who is also working as a server in a busy restaurant has probably developed excellent time-management skills and an ability to appear unflustered by unexpected situations. Another who has worked in retail may have developed an ability to calm a frustrated or dissatisfied customer through strong communication skills and by taking initiative in addressing customer complaints. Those students who are parents already know how to take responsibility for others and how to advocate for them. The list is endless. Recognizing that leadership skills in health care are no different from those required in other areas of life and acknowledging the influence of past and present life experiences can help PTAs recognize their own leadership strengths and areas in need of development.

Finally, all PTAs, whether still in school or already working in the field, need to take ownership of this expectation for leadership performance. By formally calling it "leadership" and recognizing the need for developing strong leadership traits, it can become a self-fulfilling prophecy; people often need to think of themselves as leaders before being able to demonstrate leadership abilities to others.[3] In addition, PTA program faculty, CIs, and physical therapy department supervisors and colleagues need not only to believe in this philosophy but also to share their expectations with current or future PTAs, empowering them to develop confidence in their leadership abilities by providing opportunities for skill development.

Developing PTA Leadership Skills

Leadership development starts from within oneself. **Self-reflection** is frequently cited as an essential component of leadership development.[4,7,19,22] This can be done informally, through such mechanisms as journaling, but more formal tools are also available to assist one in developing self-awareness. For example, individuals can complete one of the many questionnaires or surveys available in leadership literature, or they can have others complete questionnaires or surveys about them. These tools help individuals recognize both their areas of strength and those areas in need of further development. However self-reflection is done, most leadership experts agree that individuals must be able to lead themselves before they can effectively lead others.[4,7,22]

Once key traits are identified, how are they enhanced and further developed? Just like any other skill learned in the PTA program, leadership behaviors must be identified, practiced, and addressed through feedback that is based on witnessed performance. Research shows that students who are not given feedback on behaviors needing improvement are less likely to change those behaviors. However, many of these leadership traits fall into the category of affective behaviors, those having more to do with personality, attitudes, and feelings. The same research also shows that students are less likely to receive feedback on affective behaviors, in part because they are sometimes harder to assess or to measure.[28] However, some tools and strategies can be used to help quantify these behaviors and provide useful feedback to students.

In the Classroom

One of the best tools to use in developing leadership skills is the **"Professional Behaviors for the 21st Century"** assessment tool. As discussed in Chapter 3, this tool, developed and recently revised by the University of Wisconsin–Madison, identifies 10 traits necessary for success in physical therapy.[29,30] There are a number of similarities between these behaviors and those identified as leadership traits. Many PT and PTA programs already use this assessment tool to encourage student self-reflection and to give students feedback on these traits throughout their academic careers. By explicitly connecting these essential traits with leadership, faculty can again clarify their expectation for leadership development. By using the sample behaviors connected with the tool, students and faculty can identify specific ways in which leadership can be demonstrated and developed.

FOR REFLECTION

- Review the list of Professional Behaviors. Identify one trait that you feel is one of your strengths, and one in which you'd like to become more adept.

Professional Behaviors for the 21st Century

Critical Thinking: The ability to question logically; identify, generate and evaluate elements of logical argument; recognize and differentiate facts, appropriate or faulty inferences, and assumptions; and distinguish relevant from irrelevant information. The ability to appropriately utilize, analyze, and critically evaluate scientific evidence to develop a logical argument, and to identify and determine the impact of bias on the decision making process.

Communication Skills: The ability to communicate effectively (i.e. verbal, non-verbal, reading, writing, and listening) for varied audiences and purposes.

Problem Solving: The ability to recognize and define problems, analyze data, develop and implement solutions, and evaluate outcomes.

Interpersonal Skills: The ability to interact effectively with patients, families, colleagues, other health care professionals, and the community in a culturally aware manner.

Responsibility: The ability to be accountable for the outcomes of personal and professional actions and to follow through on commitments that encompass the profession within the scope of work, community and social responsibilities.

Professionalism: The ability to exhibit appropriate professional conduct and to represent the profession effectively while promoting the growth/development of the Physical Therapy profession.

(box continues on page 230)

Professional Behaviors for the 21st Century (continued)

Use of Constructive Feedback: The ability to seek out and identify quality sources of feedback, reflect on and integrate the feedback, and provide meaningful feedback to others.

Effective Use of Time and Resources: The ability to manage time and resources effectively to obtain the maximum possible benefit.

Stress Management: The ability to identify sources of stress and to develop and implement effective coping behaviors; this applies for interactions for: self, patients/clients and their families, members of the health care team and in work/life scenarios.

Commitment to Learning: The ability to self-direct learning to include the identification of needs and sources of learning; and to continually seek and apply new knowledge, behaviors and skills.

From May W, Kontney L, Iglarsh Z. Professional behaviors for the 21st century 2009-2010. http://www.marquette.edu/physical-therapy/documents/ProfessionalBehaviors.pdf. Accessed August 13, 2015.

Leadership can also be developed in the classroom by the way in which a student participates in various class activities. Again, leadership does not mean being the loudest, answering questions most often, or being the main spokesperson in a small-group presentation. Leadership can be demonstrated by attentive listening, thoughtful responses to questions (think quality versus quantity of responses), and a reassuring style of interaction that encourages those less confident in their skills to take risks and believe in themselves. A student who is confident in demonstrating traditional leadership traits (for example, speaking in front of a group) may need to work on taking turns in class discussions or may need to encourage less outgoing classmates to share their ideas or to go first in a group presentation. In doing so, the idea is not to turn someone into that traditional, extroverted type of leader. It is to help others to keep their unique style yet allow them to develop their initiative and confidence. These are some of the real leadership traits that are needed today, and the student who can enable others to believe in themselves is also developing invaluable skills for his own future career.[2]

This author's institution, St. Catherine University, has developed a PTA Leadership Profile, using the data collected from the program's CIs regarding entry-level behavioral expectations, to identify the leadership traits that students are expected to demonstrate by the end of their academic careers. Throughout their time in the program, students are asked to self-assess their strengths in these traits and the areas in need of additional development. Faculty and CIs also provide feedback to students regarding these behaviors during classroom activities and clinical experiences. Again, use of a tool such as this makes students aware of the expectations for leadership and gives them clear examples of how these traits are expected to be demonstrated in the clinical setting.

Leadership Profile for the St. Catherine University Entry-Level Physical Therapist Assistant

The St. Catherine University entry-level physical therapist assistant, in addition to demonstrating professional competence in skill performance, is expected to demonstrate behavioral competencies within the clinical setting. In collaboration with our Clinical Instructors (CIs), this profile has been developed to assist in standardizing the types and frequencies of behaviors that the St. Kate's entry-level PTA should demonstrate.

This profile identifies behaviors that a majority of our clinical instructors believe are most important and should be demonstrated by an entry-level PTA. It can be used as a guideline for what behaviors the student should be demonstrating consistently by the end of the final clinical experience. This tool is a guideline; it should NOT be considered an absolute standard for required performance or an all-inclusive list.

Expectations for performance may be defined differently by different CIs, in different settings. It is expected, however, that this *profile will be used by each student and CI at the start of the clinical as a mechanism for initiating discussion* about the individual site's and the student's expectations.

The St. Catherine University Entry-level PTA is expected to *consistently*:

- recognize and respond appropriately to changes in the patient's status
- manage time independently throughout the course of the day, *especially* during patient intervention sessions
- appear confident and calm (even if not feeling it inside!)
- communicate with others in a pleasant, positive manner
- manage change by demonstrating flexibility instead of stress
- prioritize responsibilities and complete tasks without reminders
- identify and initiate additional projects when assigned tasks are completed
- complete documentation on time
- teach effectively and learn enthusiastically
- make sound decisions regarding modification or progression of interventions within the patient's established plan of care
- demonstrate punctuality, reliability, and self-management

As a member of a health care team that is jointly responsible for the well being of others, the entry-level PTA is expected to demonstrate individual leadership abilities such as these listed above. He/she should also enthusiastically and willingly participate in any other designated leadership duties within the physical therapy department.

From Clynch HM. *Behavioral Expectations and Leadership Responsibilities for Entry-Level Physical Therapist Assistants* [master's thesis]. St. Paul, MN: College of St. Catherine; 2002.

Finally, using real-time practical examination testing activities may help students develop the ability to manage stress, respond quickly to changes in patient status, and manage time more effectively. As a PTA student, one may not want the additional pressure of having to demonstrate knowledge or skills while under time constraints. To avoid this added stress, PTA faculty often are inclined to provide more time for practical examinations than students would actually have in the clinic. However, without having ample opportunity to perform problem-solving and decision-making under conditions similar to that found in the clinical environment, students may not recognize their strengths or deficits in this area. Students who are able to manage stress well during real-time testing may enter their clinical experiences with increased confidence, one of those key leadership traits for which CIs are looking. Students who learn that they do not perform well under the additional stress of time constraints are able to recognize that this is a trait that needs developing; they then have the opportunity to improve on it prior to their clinical experience. These students can be encouraged to share this developmental need with their CIs, which can help the CIs to tailor the clinical experience more specifically to these students' needs.

FOR REFLECTION

- Would real-time testing be advantageous to you personally? Or would the added pressure of time in a testing situation affect how well you were able to perform?

In the Clinical Environment

Identifying a student's leadership strengths and leadership development needs before the start of a given clinical experience is extremely important. This should be done through the student's thoughtful self-reflection and in consultation with classmates and faculty, using assessment tools or other mechanisms that allow the student to be aware of his leadership development needs. Next, this assessment should be shared with the CI at the start of a clinical experience, and together, the CI and student should set goals for improving those traits during the clinical experience. Both should be proactive in seeking out opportunities for the student to practice these skills. For example, a student who needs more confidence in speaking to peers might be mentored to develop this by gradually increasing his level of participation in patient care conferences. A student who needs opportunities to improve his teaching abilities might ask to be assigned to patients whose family members need instruction in car transfers or home exercise programs. Through informal feedback and/or formal assessment mechanisms such as the Clinical Performance Instrument or other tools used by the academic program, the CI should provide feedback on the activities and on their connection to leadership traits. The student needs to be open to this feedback, again remembering that only by receiving feedback on behaviors is he likely to make necessary changes.

For PTAs starting their first job or already working in the clinic, the same process of self-identification of leadership strengths and leadership development needs can be used with their supervising PT, manager, or other supervisor. Most employers have some type of annual review process in which the PTA is asked to identify goals for development, and leadership skill is always an area that can be improved. Again, PTAs must remember that leadership is defined by behaviors and not by title or role. PTAs must lead by example, always believing in themselves and attempting to demonstrate leadership traits in every interaction with patients, families, and other providers. Some of those traits will be better developed than others, and there is no one right way to become a stronger leader. For the less experienced PTA, leadership development may be encouraged by an increasingly complex or busier caseload that allows the PTA to learn to handle gradually increasing stress and time constraints. Confidence and communication skills may be developed by additional speaking responsibilities in patient care conferences or interdisciplinary team meetings. Decision-making and problem-solving might be encouraged through participation in departmental reviews comparing achieved patient outcomes with patient goals. The PTA might be encouraged to be part of department work groups or facility-wide committees connected with safety, quality improvement, new employee orientation, or continuing education activities.

Initiative and responsibility might be facilitated by having the experienced PTA set up the department's daily schedules, track PT supervisory visits or patient's insurance reauthorization schedules, or manage day-to-day staffing needs. Both new and experienced PTAs can maintain or develop increased confidence in their knowledge base by staying on top of current evidence and intervention approaches through continuing education, participation in journal clubs, or departmental and facility in-service training opportunities. Experienced PTAs might take more of a lead role in scheduling and planning these events or seek to improve their communication skills and ability to handle stress by being presenters to their colleagues. Other leadership development might also take more traditional forms such as serving as a CI or, where allowed by law, supervising a physical therapy aide. Some PTAs, depending on their facility organization, experience, career goals, and additional educational background, may have the opportunity to move into a more formal leadership role within a rehabilitation department or a facility's administrative staff. These development opportunities for the experienced PTA are addressed more completely in Chapter 14.

In the Community

Many opportunities for leadership skill development exist within the professional community and the community at large. Opportunities for traditional leadership development through participation in the American Physical Therapy Association (APTA) are addressed in Chapters 9 and 14. However, even without taking an active formal leadership role, involvement in the local APTA chapter (whether a student or clinician) can be used to develop leadership skills. Taking part in outreach activities such as collecting items for a local food bank may enable a PTA to help develop his organizational skills. Offering to represent the chapter at a local high school science fair allows the PTA to improve his communication abilities. Attending the chapter's business meetings can help a PTA gain knowledge about current issues and threats to the profession, enabling him to return to the workplace and educate others and inspiring him to take on a more active role in advocacy or legislative issues.

If interested in developing one's leadership more formally through the APTA, the Health Policy and Administration Section's Institute for Leadership Development has developed a **Leadership, Administration, Management, and Professionalism (LAMP) certificate program.** This series of courses and structured activities is designed to help PTs and PTAs develop their leadership skills through self-assessment, goal development, and mentoring.[31]

Within the greater community in which PTAs live, there are numerous opportunities for leadership skill development. For students, given all of the demands currently placed on them by academic programs, employers, and families, having time for additional commitments may seem impossible. This may be an area that remains untapped until such time as students have completed their PTA education. Conversely, places of worship, schools, and other volunteer organizations can often use assistance for small or short-term commitments. Taking on these types of tasks may be less daunting yet will still enable a student to demonstrate leadership skills such as initiative, responsibility, and the ability to multitask. In addition, adding this to a résumé and being able to articulate how it helped develop leadership traits may put a student in a more marketable position upon graduation.

SUMMARY

Thinking of themselves as leaders, especially within the context of physical therapy, may be a different mind-set for both PTA students and working PTAs. Needing and encouraging PTA leadership may also be a different way of thinking for many PTs. However, by looking at leadership in a nontraditional sense and connecting today's definition of leadership with the current needs of the health-care environment, it is clear that leadership should be an expectation for every PTA. By recognizing this while a student and taking ownership of this expectation, future PTAs are in the best position to use classroom, clinical, and community opportunities to develop their leadership behaviors. This will enable them to transition into the leadership expectations of the work environment with greatest ease.

REFERENCES

1. American Physical Therapy Association. *A Normative Model of Physical Therapist Assistant Education: Version 2007.* Alexandria, VA: American Physical Therapy Association; 2007.
2. Hayhurst C. A time to lead: leadership programs in physical therapy. *PT in Motion.* 2010;2(7):14-21.
3. McConnell CR. *The Effective Health Care Supervisor.* 8th ed. Gaithersburg, MD: Aspen; 2015:589.
4. Northouse P. *Leadership: Theory and Practice.* 6th ed. New Delhi, India: Sage Publications; 2013.
5. Kotter J. *Force for Change: How Leadership Differs From Management.* New York, NY: Simon & Schuster Free Press; 1990.
6. Dye CF. *Leadership in Healthcare: Values at the Top.* Chicago, IL: Health Administration Press; 2000:234-671.

7. Kouzes JM, Posner BZ. *The Leadership Challenge.* 5th ed. San Francisco, CA: Jossey-Bass; 2012:394.

8. Levey S, Hill J, Greene B. Leadership in health care and the leadership literature. *J Ambulatory Care Manag.* 2002;25(2):68-74.

9. Wang MC, Hyun JK, Harrison MI, Shortell SM, Fraser I. Redesigning health systems for quality: lessons from emerging practices. *Jt Comm J Qual Saf.* 2006;32(11):599-611.

10. Sanders B. A team approach: leadership in physical therapy education. *J Phys Ther Educ.* 1998;12(3):21-24.

11. Garcia VH, Meek KL, Wilson KA. Advancing innovation in health care leadership: a collaborative experience. *Nurs Adm Q.* 2011;35(3):242.

12. VanDeusen Lukas C, Holmes SK, Cohen AB, et al. Transformational change in health care systems: an organizational model. *Health Care Manag Rev.* 2007; 32(4):309-320.

13. Lawrence D. *From Chaos to Care: The Promise of Team-Based Medicine.* Cambridge, MA: Da Capo Press; 2002:185.

14. Issacson N. Leadership, accountability and wellness in organizations. *J Phys Ther Educ.* 1998;12(3):18-20.

15. Lee T, Mongan J. *Chaos and Organization in Health Care.* Cambridge, MA: MIT Press; 2009:380.

16. Shortell SM. Increasing value: a research agenda for addressing the managerial and organizational challenges facing health care delivery in the United States. *Med Care Res Rev 2004.* 2004;61(12S).

17. de Zulueta P. Developing compassionate leadership in health care: an integrative review. *J Heathc Leadersh.* 2015;2016(8):1-10.

18. Glickman SW, Baggett KA, Krubert CG, Peterson ED, Schulman KA. Promoting quality: the health care organization from a management perspective. *Int J Qual Health Care.* 2007;19(6):341-348.

19. MacPhee M, Chang L, Lee D, Spiri W. Global health care leadership development: trends to consider. *J Heathc Leadersh.* 2013;5:21+.

20. Schmoll BJ. Educational leadership from a holistic perspective. *J Phys Ther Educ.* 1998;12(3):6-17.

21. El-Din D. Leadership: a focus on what matters. *J Phys Ther Educ.* 1998;12(3): 25-27.

22. Dye CF, Garman AN. *Exceptional Leadership: 16 Critical Competencies for Healthcare Executives.* 2nd ed. Chicago, IL: Health Administration Press; 2014.

23. Woods E. Opportunity out of adversity: physical therapy's unique legacy. *PT Magazine.* 2002;10(9):46-52.

24. Mathwig K, Clarke F, Owens T, Gramet P. Selection criteria for employment of entry-level physical therapists: a survey of New York State employers. *J Phys Ther Educ.* 2001;15(1):65-74.

25. Clynch HM. *Behavioral Expectations and Leadership Responsibilities for Entry-Level Physical Therapist Assistants* [master's thesis]. St. Paul, MN: College of St. Catherine; 2002.

26. Rogers R. Leadership communication styles: a descriptive analysis of health care professionals. *J Healthc Leadersh.* 2012;2012(4):47-57.

27. Solberg JJ. Lessons in leadership. *PT Magazine*. 2008;16(7):42-44.
28. Hayes KW, Huber H, Rogers J, Sanders B. Behaviors that cause clinical instructors to question the clinical competence of physical therapist students. *Phys Ther*. 1999;79:653-671.
29. May WW, Morgan BJ, Lemke JC, Karst GM, Stone HL. Model for ability-based assessment in physical therapy education. *J Phys Ther Educ*. 1995;9(1):3-6.
30. May W, Kontney L, Iglarsh Z. Professional behaviors for the 21st century 2009-2010. http://www.marquette.edu/physical-therapy/documents/ProfessionalBehaviors.pdf. Accessed August 13, 2015.
31. APTA Health Policy and Administration Section. LAMP leadership development certificate program. The Institute for Leadership in Physical Therapy Web site. http://www.aptahpa.org/?page=57. Updated 2015. Accessed October 17, 2015.

Name _____

REVIEW

1. In your own words, define what leadership means.

_____

_____

_____

_____

2. Do you believe that leadership is different from management? Defend your answer.

_____

_____

_____

_____

3. In your opinion, what leadership traits are most essential for you as a PTA to demonstrate?

_____

_____

_____

_____

(questions continue on page 238)

Application

1. Identify two leadership traits that you feel you already possess. Describe how you demonstrate each of these traits.

   _____

   _____

   _____

   _____

2. Identify two leadership traits that you feel you need to develop. Explain why you have difficulty in demonstrating each of these behaviors.

   _____

   _____

   _____

   _____

3. Using the following table, begin a plan for leadership skill development.

Leadership Behaviors That Need Further Development:	Ideas for Working on Trait in the *Classroom/Continuing Education:*	Ideas for Working on Trait in the *Clinical Setting:*	Ideas for Working on Trait in the *Professional or Local Community:*	Time Frame for Development/Other Resources Needed to Assist in Development:

13

Evidence-Based Practice and Research Review Fundamentals

CHAPTER OBJECTIVES

After reading this chapter, the reader will be able to:

- Define evidence-based practice (EBP).
- Describe the principles on which EBP is based.
- Discuss how EBP is used to support the delivery of physical therapy services.
- Describe the role of the physical therapist assistant (PTA) in EBP.
- Identify various resources for obtaining and using clinical evidence.
- Compare and contrast the various levels of evidence.
- Describe how clinical research supports the use of EBP.
- Define various terms related to research methodology.
- Describe basic techniques for critically appraising a research article.

KEY TERMS AND CONCEPTS

- Evidence-based practice (EBP)
- PICO question (patient, intervention, control or comparison, outcome)
- Clinical practice guidelines
- Levels of evidence
- Abstract
- Literature review
- Hypothesis
- Randomized controlled trial (RCT)
- Single vs. double blinding/masking
- Experimental/control group
- Critically appraised topic (CAT)

Jessica and Khaliq, two PTAs working in an outpatient setting, are discussing some of the various physical agents that they have been using while working with clients with low back pain. Jessica mentions that the physical therapist (PT) with whom she is teamed does not generally include many physical agents in her plans of care, relying almost exclusively on manual therapy and exercise for her intervention programs. Jessica states that the PT says there isn't enough evidence

(vignette continues on page 242)

to support the use of most physical agents during physical therapy. Khaliq responds that his supervising PT uses some type of thermal modality with almost every client who reports chronic low back pain, telling Khaliq that she gets a better response to manual therapy and exercise after the use of heat. Jessica and Khaliq wonder why their supervising PTs have such different approaches and are interested in determining which PT's approach is more effective.

QUESTIONS TO CONSIDER

What is meant by the term "evidence"? How do we go about finding evidence to support what is done in the clinical setting? Are some types of evidence better than others? What is the PTA's role in obtaining and using evidence? How do we critically appraise a research article? What are some of the ways in which PTs and PTAs share their knowledge of evidence with each other?

Physical therapy has progressed from a field in which decisions regarding interventions were made by the physician to a profession in which the PT has become an autonomous practitioner. Along with this progression toward independent practice has come PTs' increased responsibility to justify their decision-making processes.[1] In addition, third-party payers have become more selective in what types of interventions they will pay for and have started to ask for more proof regarding the efficacy of many of the interventions that PTs and PTAs perform. It is no longer enough for the clinician to base her use of a particular technique on the results she has obtained using it in the past or on a theoretical model of what effects it might have. Today's clinicians are expected to implement interventions that are based on results supported by scientific literature, following a protocol called "evidence-based practice."

Evidence-based practice (EBP) has its roots in the medical community, where it was called "evidence-based medicine."[2] Although the philosophy of using evidence to support medical decisions goes back as far as the mid-1800s,[3] it was only in the 1990s that the directives for using the process of EBP first began to appear in physical therapy literature.[1] EBP has been defined by Sackett et al as "the conscientious, explicit, and judicious use of current best evidence in making decisions about the care of individual patients . . . integrating individual clinical expertise with the best available external clinical evidence from systematic research."[3] The second part of that definition is an important component of the effective use of EBP. Although the use of the best available evidence should be incorporated into the PT's decision-making regarding intervention protocols, operating in an EBP manner also includes the clinician reflecting on her own clinical expertise and ability to recognize individual patient/client needs and preferences.[4] For example, the literature might indicate that ultrasound delivered concurrently with other interventions improves the outcomes of patients who are being treated for a

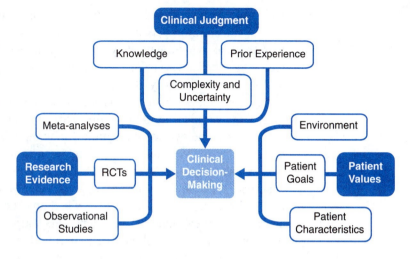

Figure 13-1 The three components of evidence-based practice, including research evidence, clinical judgment, and patient values, should be viewed in relation to their contributions to clinical decision-making. (Reprinted with permission from Portney, LG. Evidence-based practice and clinical decision making: it's not just the research course anymore. *J Phys Ther Educ*. 2004;18[3]:46–51.)

particular diagnosis. However, if a particular patient reports to the clinician a high level of anxiety about receiving ultrasound because of a previous negative experience with it, the clinician might appropriately choose not to include it in the plan of care. Although it is important to make decisions on the basis of science whenever possible, EBP is not a "cookbook" with specific directions that must be followed. Portney (Fig. 13-1) states that "evidence-based decision-making" may be a more appropriate term to use for the process, as it reflects the clinician's ability to integrate the available evidence along with her clinical expertise and experience and the uniqueness of each patient's situation when making clinical decisions.[4]

The PTA's Role in EBP

A PTA reading this text might be thinking, "Why is it important that I understand the principles of EBP? I am not going to be developing the patient's plan of care. That is the PT's role." It is true that a PTA is not expected to use current evidence in the same manner as does a PT. For example, the recent revision of the American Physical Therapy Association's (APTA's) Code of Ethics for the Physical Therapist includes a standard that requires PTs to incorporate evidence into their professional judgments, whereas the corresponding section of the Standards of Ethical Conduct for the Physical Therapist Assistant does not mention evidence, only "best practice."[5,6] However, according to the Commission on Accreditation for Physical Therapy Education (CAPTE), entry-level PTAs should be expected to read a research article, identify the various sections of the article, describe the type of content found in each section, and synthesize the relevant information as it applies to their clinical work, all as part of the problem-solving process.[7] A PTA should be able to articulate an understanding of why one intervention might be used rather than another.

Although it may not be appropriate for the PTA to discuss why a particular intervention was or was not included on a patient's plan of care, PTAs should always seek to expand their already-strong knowledge base related to the rationale for an intervention and should be able to discuss the evidence that supports the use of one type of intervention versus another. Patients sometimes may ask the PTA working with them to explain why they are receiving certain interventions or why they aren't receiving other interventions that they may have received in the past. If the PTA is unable to verbalize why she is providing a given intervention, she runs the risk of being seen as a provider who is merely doing what she is told to do, lacking judgment or critical-thinking skills. This perception could diminish the PTA's credibility in the eyes of the patient (or supervising PT). Conversely, the PTA who is up to date with current evidence and can share that knowledge appropriately may be perceived as more effective and more competent. As a PTA develops clinical expertise, especially if she sees a given patient more frequently than the PT, she may be in a better position to recognize when an ordered intervention is not effective or appropriate, even though the evidence may support its use. By understanding the principles of how EBP should be paired with clinical expertise, the PTA is able to report her observations to the PT with greater confidence and is better equipped to participate in a discussion of alternatives or other approaches. Finally, by understanding how to seek and find the highest quality of evidence, the PTA can team with the PT in the formal process of seeking answers.

Developing the Question

Either a PT or a PTA can initiate the first component of EBP, which is the development of a question relating to a patient/client situation. A clinician is not considered to be following EBP if she merely looks for an article that supports the use of a particular intervention she has included on a care plan. Rather, the process of EBP should be entered with the assumption that the answer to the question isn't already known.[8] To make a clinical question more open and less biased toward one outcome or another, experts in EBP recommend using the acronym **PICO** to help shape the components of a clinical question. PICO stands for:[8–11]

- **Patient:** A description of the patient diagnosis to which the clinician would apply the answer to the question
- **Intervention:** The procedure the clinician is studying
- **Control (or Comparison):** Those who do not receive the intervention or receive a different intervention
- **Outcome:** The results that the clinician would like to see achieved by the patient

Using this format helps the clinician to more easily determine whether the results of available research can be applied to a specific patient population.

FOR REFLECTION

- Go back to the scenario at the beginning of the chapter. Based on the information provided there, could you write an appropriate PICO question to attempt to answer Jessica and Khaliq's question? Why or why not? What additional information might be helpful in writing your question?

Finding the Evidence

Once a clinician has established a PICO question, where and how should she begin to look for the answers? Various groups, including the APTA, have attempted to assist clinicians in using EBP by developing **clinical practice guidelines.** These guidelines may be related to a specific diagnosis, as in the APTA Orthopaedic Section's clinical practice guidelines for neck pain,[12] or to the use of a specific intervention used to treat a diagnosis, such as the Ottawa Panel's guidelines for the use of therapeutic exercise for patients with fibromyalgia.[13] Clinical practice guidelines consolidate the current evidence available on a topic, enabling the clinician to deliver interventions in a manner that follows currently recommended best practice. Unfortunately, most clinical situations involve diagnoses or patient situations that are not covered by current clinical practice guidelines. The clinician then must search on her own for the answers.

In years past, many clinicians used the challenges of finding and reviewing literature as a rationale for not practicing in an evidence-based manner.[14] The advent of the Internet and the development of numerous databases that categorize medical literature have alleviated the difficulty in finding the literature,[11] but the volume of information now available to clinicians can be overwhelming and, in its own way, can also interfere with the use of evidence.[14] Having the time to search for evidence has been noted in multiple studies as a barrier to implementing EBP.[2,15,16] However, familiarity with the most common medical search engines and the ways in which searches can be made more precise can make the research associated with EBP much more efficient.[15] Each database has specific procedures that can be used to focus a search. A detailed description of how to most effectively use every database available is beyond the scope of this text; however, a few strategies are universal to most of the commonly used databases:

- Search multiple databases at once, whenever possible.
- Use an "advanced search" feature, which allows use of more specific search terms.
- Combine search terms using the components of the PICO question. For example, instead of searching for "ultrasound," a search might connect "ultrasound," "pain," "knee," and "osteoarthritis." Some databases recommend using certain search terms. In PubMed, these are called "MeSH" (medical subject heading) terms, and although it isn't necessary to use them, doing so will make a search most efficient.[8]
- Use "limits" to make the search more specific, such as searching for articles in English only (unless one can read in other languages), in a particular type of study format, in relation to a certain component of patient/client management (i.e., "intervention" rather than "diagnosis"), and published in a particular time frame, among many other types of limits or "subsets" of search terms.

FOR REFLECTION
FOR REFLECTION

- Identify at least two search terms and one search limit that would increase the effectiveness of a search for evidence related to the scenario presented at the beginning of the chapter.

Students generally have free access to a number of databases through their academic institution's library website. Once out of school, clinicians can access multiple databases through their APTA membership. All members have access to PTNow, a website developed by APTA for the purpose of quickly disseminating evidence for clinical use. At the site, clinicians have access to multiple databases and medical journals, as well as clinical practice guidelines, clinical summaries (information related to patient/client management of a certain condition), and databases compiled by various APTA sections.[17]

For more detailed information on how to best use the specific databases to which a student or clinician has access, the best resource may be a professional librarian at your academic institution, work setting or clinical site (if it has a medical library), or local library branch.[18] Table 13-1 summarizes a number of different evidence-based databases.

Assessing the Evidence

How do we determine what qualifies as "current best evidence"? Some types of research are considered to be stronger evidence than others. The ranking of different types of research, called hierarchies or **levels of evidence,** may vary somewhat, depending on the type of clinical question being answered (for example, a question related to diagnosis versus one related to use of an intervention).[3,8] Table 13-2 is a compilation of the general categorical levels found in many of the hierarchies of evidence related to intervention.[8–10]

Reading a Research Article

Once articles are located, the PTA must be able to interpret the information within them. The following discussion is designed to provide a basic familiarity with the format commonly used in articles related to effectiveness of interventions (which is probably the type of research article most relevant to PTAs). It also includes brief definitions of the terminology that might be found within each section of an article. For more in-depth information on research terminology and methodology, look to the textbooks referenced at the end of this chapter from which these definitions are taken.[8,19–21]

Abstract

The **abstract** is found at the beginning of an article (in addition, it may be the only part of an article that is available through certain online database searches). Usually only one to two paragraphs long, the abstract gives a very brief description of the purpose, methods, outcomes, and importance of the study. Another format of an

(text continues on page 248)

Table 13-1   Examples of Evidence-Based Databases[8,17,18]

Database	Publisher	Web Address	Free?	Other Information
CINAHL (Cumulative Index to Nursing and Allied Health Literature)	EBSCO Publishing	www.cinahl.com	No	Includes some PT section journals that may not be accessible via other free search engines
Cochrane Library	The Cochrane Collaboration	www.thecochranelibrary.com	Yes	Includes a number of databases, including one specifically for systematic reviews
PEDro (Physiotherapy Evidence Database)	University of Sydney, Australia	www.pedro.org.au/	Yes	Focused on physical therapy research; articles are rated for validity and ease of data interpretation
PTNow	American Physical Therapy Association	www.PTNow.org	Yes to APTA members. In addition, some section journals can only be accessed with section membership	Includes links to clinical practice guidelines, clinical summaries, and outcome tests and measures
PubMed/ MEDLINE	U.S. National Library of Medicine/ National Institutes of Health	www.ncbi.nlm.nih.gov/ PubMed/	Yes, but access to articles may not be	Does not provide full text articles but does provide links to some of them

Table 13-2 Hierarchy of Evidence for Intervention (From Highest to Lowest)[8,9]

Type of Evidence[8,20,21]	Description[8,20,21]
Systematic reviews/ meta-analyses	Systematic reviews analyze multiple studies already performed in a subject area, classifying them in terms of quality and outcomes. Meta-analyses compare the same variable studied in multiple articles in an attempt to quantify the results.
Randomized controlled trials	A study in which subjects are randomly assigned either to an experimental group that receives a given intervention or to a control group that receives no intervention. Outcomes of the experimental group are then compared with those of the control group.
"All or none" studies	Subjects all responded negatively before a given intervention is provided, but only some do so after receiving it, OR some subjects responded negatively before a given intervention is provided, but now none do after receiving it.
Cohort studies	One or more groups of similar subjects are followed over a period of time to see whether differences develop based on exposure to another variable.
Case control studies	Subjects for a study are selected based on having a particular condition; they are then retroactively studied to determine whether there were other common factors that predisposed them to that condition.
Case series studies	Comparing a few individuals with similar individual presentations or outcomes.
Individual case studies	One patient's history, condition, and outcomes are analyzed.
Expert opinion/ experience	Using an intervention because of past success in using it or because of someone else's recommendation.

abstract can currently be found when accessing the electronic format of *Physical Therapy*, the journal of the APTA. Each month's edition is accompanied by an online podcast in which the journal's editor-in-chief summarizes each article's methodology, results, and "bottom line" implications for clinical practice.[22]

Introduction

Most studies begin with some background information to explain why the research to be presented was necessary. This includes a **literature review,** a summary of relevant research that has been previously performed on the topic, and the gaps that are present in current research. The authors then address the purpose of the study, identifying what they hoped to learn from it. They may explicitly state a **hypothesis,** in which they predict the outcome of the study in terms of how the variables studied are connected. One version of this, in which the author predicts there will be no difference between variables in a study, is called a null hypothesis.

Methods

The methods section should identify the type of study that was performed (cohort study, systematic review, etc.). As noted in Table 13-2, the **randomized controlled trial (RCT),** also known as randomized clinical trial or randomized controlled clinical trial, is highest on the hierarchy of evidence among individual studies (systematic reviews and meta-analyses look at multiple studies). In an RCT, subjects in the study should be assigned to one of two (or sometimes more) groups that receive different forms or combinations of interventions (or no intervention). The bigger the groups, the more likely it is that the groups are truly comparable (and that any difference in results is not related to chance).[21] The way in which the subjects are put into these groups should be described and should indeed be random, performed in a manner that ensures as much similarity between the groups as possible and minimizes the chance of any bias influencing the makeup of the groups. Often this process is performed by a computer or in some other structured way (a coin flip, etc.) by someone who will not be involved with the rest of the study to keep the researchers or subjects unaware of the group to which each subject has been assigned. This lack of awareness is known as **blinding** or **masking.** When only one group (the subjects or the researchers) is unaware of the categorization, this is referred to as a **single-blind** study; in a **double-blind** study, neither is aware of how subjects are grouped.[8,18]

A group receiving an intervention being studied is considered an **experimental group,** and a group that receives no intervention is called a **control group.** Sometimes a control group is given a sham intervention, an intervention that does not have an effect (such as an ultrasound intervention being delivered via a machine that has been altered so that sound waves are not transmitted), to blind the subjects as to which group they actually belong.

FOR REFLECTION

FOR REFLECTION

- Why is it important for researchers to be blinded to the subjects' group assignments? Why do the subjects themselves often need to be blinded?

Some studies will use a comparison group instead of a control group and will look at the effectiveness of one intervention versus another, but without a control group it is difficult to say with certainty that either intervention made a difference because the patients may have improved even without receiving any intervention. Unfortunately, control groups are not always used. In some cases, it is known that failing to provide a proven intervention for a patient (such as a type of medication) would not be in the patient's best interests, and therefore it would be unethical to have a control group.

Table 13-3   Additional Terms Related to Research Methodology[8,19,20]

Term	Definition
Convenience sample	A subgroup of the population that can be more easily studied, for instance, all patients with brain tumors admitted to a given hospital in a given year.
Dependent variable	The end result being compared between the two groups after receiving (or not receiving) the intervention. In studies related to physical therapy interventions, it is often related to some change in function or relief of pain.
Independent variable	The intervention being studied or manipulated by the researcher; in other words, it is what makes the experimental group different from the control group.
N	The number of participants in a study or within a given group. Often written as $N =$ (the number).
Population	The overall group or subject matter being studied, for instance, patients with brain tumors. Usually impossible to study every subject in the population.

Performing research in an ethical manner includes making subjects aware of the potential risks of participating in a research study, and whenever possible, the risks of participation should be minimized. Some studies will have one group receive an intervention and the other group receive the same intervention plus an additional one and will attempt to compare the results; but again, without a pure control group, erroneous assumptions could be made. Potential studies are generally required to be reviewed and approved by a facility's institutional review board, which, among other responsibilities, monitors the procedures of a study to ensure that subjects are protected from harm.[23] Table 13-3 notes some additional terms relevant to research methodology.

Results

The goal of the results section is usually to show whether or not the use of the independent variable (the intervention being studied) made any difference in the results, measured by the dependent variable. However, it is not enough just to be able to show differences in the data collected. A researcher must be able to prove the statistical significance of the data: the researcher must use statistical measures to verify that the results did not occur by chance.

The different types of statistics included in research articles are intimidating and confusing to many clinicians, who often don't understand how they were calculated or what they mean.[8] Descriptive statistics are those that summarize the characteristics and distribution of the data collected. Parametric and nonparametric statistics use mathematical formulas that attempt to establish relationships or differences between sets of data. Different statistical tests are used depending on the way the data are collected and their type. It is often more important to understand what a particular statistical term is assessing or representing than it is to know exactly how to calculate the statistic itself.[8,18] Clinicians must remember that statistics can often be manipulated or presented in ways that are more favorable than others, and a study that has few statistical tests included is likely to have questionable validity.[18] Conversely, the more favorable statistics there are associated with a certain outcome, the more likely it is that the results are accurate.[8] Table 13-4 discusses some additional terms related to research results and analysis.

Discussion

A discussion section may follow the presentation of the statistical data. In this section, the authors share their thoughts on why they obtained the results that they did, along with the clinical implications of the study results. The authors will often compare the results they obtained with those obtained in the studies addressed in the literature review at the beginning of the article. If their study involved using a particular assessment tool or functional outcome measure, the authors may compare the results they obtained with studies using similar tools that purportedly measure the same outcome, to make a recommendation regarding which tool might be best for a given clientele.

Within this section, or sometimes in a separate one called "Limitations," the researchers will identify any factors that may have contributed to inaccuracy or unreliability of the results, may have contributed to results not being statistically significant, or may have interfered with the study being conducted as objectively as possible. One common limitation is a small number of participants; as stated previously, with larger study groups it is easier to prove that results are due to a true difference and not just to chance. Another common limitation is the inability to blind the subjects about which study group they were assigned. Table 13-5 lists terms related to research tools and outcome measures.

Conclusion

In the conclusion of the article, the researchers will usually again summarize the purpose of the study, the results, and the reasons the results of the study are important. Often they will identify future studies that could be performed to build on their results or to improve on any methodology issues that may have interfered with the reliability of their results.

Table 13-4   Terms Related to Research Results and Analysis[8,18,21]

Term	Definition
Confidence interval	The probability that a true score for a variable lies between a certain range of scores. Generally expected to be at 95% or more.
Effect size	Compares the difference between two means, usually represented by a number between 0 and 1. A higher score indicates a greater amount of difference, with 0.2 representing minimal effect, 0.5 as moderate, and 0.8 as a large effect.
Intent to treat	A number that includes all subjects (even those who are noncompliant or drop out) in the final analysis of data. Preserves randomization. Studies that do not provide dropout data could possibly be biased.
Mean	The average of all responses/scores in a set of data.
Median	The middle response/score in a set of numerical data. If there is an even number of scores, the median is the average between the middle two.
Mode	The most common response/score in a set of data.
Number needed to treat	The minimum number of subjects needed to receive an experimental intervention to get one favorable result (or reduce risk of a negative one). A smaller number is better.
Outlier	A score that is unusually higher or lower than the other scores in the same data set.
Probability	The likelihood that the results of the study could have occurred by chance (not because of a real difference in interventions). Usually a P value of 0.05 or less is required for the results to be considered statistically significant.
Skewness	Occurs when the mean is affected by the presence of one or more outliers; a mean that is positively skewed is made higher by an outlier, whereas negative skewness means the mean is brought down.
Standard deviation	The amount by which scores vary from the mean. A higher standard deviation means there is more variation in scores.

Table 13-5   Terms Related to Research Tools and Outcome Measures[8,19]

Term	Definition
Instrument reliability	The consistency with which a measurement tool gives the same result with repeated use. There are various ways of demonstrating this.
Inter-rater reliability	The consistency of scores in the same measurements taken by multiple clinicians.
Intra-rater reliability	The consistency of scores taken by one clinician taken at different times.
Sensitivity	A test's ability to identify people who have a certain condition. High sensitivity means there are very few times when someone who doesn't have the condition will actually test positive for it (a "false positive").
Specificity	A test's ability to identify people who do not have a certain condition. High specificity means there are very few times when someone who has the condition actually tests negative for it (a "false negative").
Validity	The ability of a measurement tool to measure what it is supposed to measure. There are many types of measurement validity.

Sharing the Evidence

Once the clinician has reviewed the evidence and found answers, she must be able to share that information with others. One format for doing so was developed by the original practitioners of evidence-based medicine and is called a **critically appraised topic (CAT).** A CAT is a brief review of the evidence found related to the PICO question. If written in relation to one particular study, a CAT may be as short as one page. CATs that present evidence compiled from multiple articles on a given subject may be slightly longer. Results are usually presented in very concise formats, often using tables or charts, and are summarized in a one- or two-line "clinical bottom line."[9] The Centre for Evidence-Based Medicine has a free software download, CATMaker, which assists clinicians in researching and developing a CAT.[10,14] Regardless of whether or not they are presented in the format of a CAT, results of PICO-based searches are often shared with colleagues through informal "journal clubs" (regularly scheduled meetings to discuss current research), departmental staff meetings, or formal presentations with clinicians from multiple departments within a facility.

PTAs may also be involved in EPB through participation in the creation of original research. The ways that PTAs commonly participate in research and the mechanisms they might use to share the results of that research are addressed in Chapter 14.

SUMMARY

Although the majority of PTs believe in the necessity of following EBP, most of them also agree that they need to increase their own use of evidence.[2] Clinical experience, although a component of evidence-based practice, is still being used more often than clinical research by a significant number of both experienced and novice clinicians, though newer graduates appear to have better skills in finding current evidence.[24] PTAs need to be able to use current evidence to explain to patients why and how they are delivering interventions. Those PTAs who are familiar with the principles of EBP, who can efficiently access clinical databases, and who can understand basic research methodology and terminology will be in a better position to support the incorporation of high-quality evidence into clinical practice.

REFERENCES

1. Schreiber J, Stern P. A review of the literature on evidence-based practice in physical therapy. *Internet J Allied Health Sci Pract*. 2005;3(4):17.
2. Jette DU, Bacon K, Batty C, et al. Evidence-based practice: beliefs, attitudes, knowledge, and behaviors of physical therapists. *Phys Ther*. 2003;83(9):786-805.
3. Sackett DL, Rosenberg WMC, Muir Gray, JA, Haynes RB, Richardson, WS. Evidence based medicine: what it is and what it isn't. *BMJ*. 1996;312(7023):71-72.
4. Portney LG. Evidence-based practice and clinical decision making: it's not just the research course anymore. *J Phys Ther Educ*. 2004;18(3):46-51.
5. American Physical Therapy Association. Code of ethics for the physical therapist. http://www.apta.org/uploadedFiles/APTAorg/About_Us/Policies/Ethics/CodeofEthics.pdf. Updated 2009. Accessed August 22, 2015.
6. American Physical Therapy Association. Standards of ethical conduct for the physical therapist assistant. http://www.apta.org/uploadedFiles/APTAorg/About_Us/Policies/Ethics/StandardsEthicalConductPTA.pdf. Updated 2015. Accessed August 13, 2015.
7. American Physical Therapy Association. *A Normative Model of Physical Therapist Assistant Education: Version 2007*. Alexandria, VA: American Physical Therapy Association; 2007.
8. Jewell D. *Guide to Evidence-Based Physical Therapy Practice*. 2nd ed. Sudbury, MA: Jones & Bartlett; 2011.
9. Straus SE, Glasziou P, Richardson WS, Haynes RB. *Evidence-Based Medicine: How to Practice and Teach It*. 4th ed. Philadelphia, PA: Elsevier Churchill Livingstone; 2011.

10. University of Oxford. Centre for Evidence-Based Medicine. http://www.cebm.net. Updated 2014. Accessed September 5, 2015.

11. Slavin MD. Teaching evidence-based practice in physical therapy: critical competencies and necessary conditions. *J Phys Ther Educ*. 2004;18(3):4-11.

12. Childs JD, Cleland JA, Elliott JM, et al. Neck pain. *J Orthop Sports Phys Ther*. 2008;38(9):A1-A34.

13. Brosseau L, Wells GA, Tugwell P, et al. Ottawa Panel Evidence-Based Clinical Practice Guidelines for aerobic fitness exercises in the management of fibromyalgia: part 1. *Phys Ther*. 2008;88(7):857-871.

14. Fell DW, Burnham JB. Access is key: teaching students and physical therapists to access evidence, expert opinion, and patient values for evidence-based practice. *J Phys Ther Educ*. 2004;18(3):12-23.

15. Richter RR, Austin TM. Using MeSH (medical subject headings) to enhance PubMed search strategies for evidence-based practice in physical therapy. *Phys Ther*. 2012;92(1):124-132.

16. Ramírez-Vélez R, Bagur-Calafat MC, Correa-Bautista JE, Girabent-Farrés M. Barriers against incorporating evidence-based practice in physical therapy in Colombia: current state and factors associated. *BMC Med Educ*. 2015;15(1):220.

17. American Physical Therapy Association. PTNow. PTNow.org. Updated 2015. Accessed October 10, 2015.

18. Greenhalgh T. *How to Read a Paper: The Basics of Evidence-Based Medicine*. 4th ed. Oxford, England: Wiley-Blackwell; 2010.

19. Portney LG, Watkins MP. *Foundations of Clinical Research: Applications to Practice*. 3rd ed. Upper Saddle River, NJ: Pearson/Prentice-Hall; 2009.

20. Carter R, Lubinsky J, Domholdt E. *Rehabilitation Research: Principles and Applications*. 4th ed. St. Louis, MO: Elsevier Saunders; 2011.

21. Herbert R, Jamtvedt G, Birger Hagen K, Mead J. *Practical Evidence-Based Physiotherapy*. 2nd ed. London, England: Elsevier Churchill Livingstone; 2011.

22. American Physical Therapy Association. PTJ podcast central. http://ptjournal.apta.org/site/misc/podcasts.xhtml#craikcast. Updated 2015. Accessed October 10, 2015.

23. St. Catherine University. Institutional review board. https://www2.stkate.edu/IRB/home. Updated 2015. Accessed October 10, 2015.

24. Manns PJ, Norton AV, Darrah J. Cross-sectional study to examine evidence-based practice skills and behaviors of physical therapy graduates: is there a knowledge-to-practice gap? *Phys Ther*. 2015;95(4):568-578.

Name _____

REVIEW

1. Define the term "evidence-based practice."

_____

_____

_____

_____

2. How does EBP take the patient's wishes into consideration?

_____

_____

_____

_____

3. What is the highest type of evidence found on the hierarchy of evidence for intervention? Why is this type of evidence higher than the others?

_____

_____

_____

_____

4. Differentiate between the following terms:

■ Dependent variable/independent variable

_____

_____

(questions continue on page 258)

- Mode/median/mean

_____

_____

- Validity/reliability

_____

_____

Application

1. Write a PICO question related to the scenario at the beginning of this chapter. Be as specific as possible with your question (for example, you may choose a particular spinal diagnosis instead of using "chronic low back pain").

P: _____

I: _____

C: _____

O: _____

2. Using the PICO question in number 1 (or another of your own choosing), search for evidence in two of the databases listed in this chapter. Compare the results of the two searches.

Databases used: _____

_____

Did both searches yield the same number of articles? _____

If the answer to this question is no, why do you think there was a difference?

_____

_____

_____

_____

14

Beginning Your Career, Post-Graduation Advanced Learning, and Skill Development

After reading this chapter, the reader will be able to:

- Explain why taking advantage of continuing education (CE) and career development opportunities is essential for a successful career as a physical therapist assistant (PTA).
- Discuss the opportunities for career development related to serving as a clinical instructor (CI).
- Identify roles that the PTA may hold in the clinical setting outside that of direct patient care.
- Identify the roles that PTAs may serve in physical therapy education programs.
- Identify routes for continuing formal education and obtaining additional academic degrees within and outside of physical therapy.
- Describe mechanisms for identifying and recognizing advanced skills through the American Physical Therapy Association (APTA).
- Describe potential ways in which PTAs may participate in performing and presenting research.
- Explain the purpose of the PTA Advanced Proficiency Pathways (APPs).
- Describe the mechanism for becoming more involved in the APTA at a national level.

KEY TERMS AND CONCEPTS

- Jurisprudence examination
- Clinical instructor (CI)
- Continuing education (CE)
- Degree completion programs
- In-service
- Case study
- Poster presentation
- Platform presentation
- Recognition of Advanced Proficiency for the Physical Therapist Assistant
- Advanced Proficiency Pathways (APPs)
- New Professionals
- Sections
- Special interest groups (SIGs)

Agroup of second-year students in a local PTA program have gathered for their capstone seminar and are discussing their future plans after graduation, only a few weeks away. Ryan states, "I can't wait to be done with school. I can't believe that this is the last college class that I am ever going to take!" Hassan says, "Really? I know I will be going back to school someday." Sarah responds to Hassan, "I didn't know you were planning on becoming a physical therapist someday. I am, too! That's cool!" Hassan replies, "I'm not sure that I want to become a PT, but I know that I'll want to do something to build on my PTA skills." Ryan asks him, "But how else would you do that, other than going back to school to become a PT?" Ryan then turns to Sarah and asks, "Does being a PTA mean you don't have to take as many classes when you go back to school to become a PT?"

QUESTIONS TO CONSIDER

What are other educational options for those who want to build on their PTA skills? Are there other ways, beyond returning to school, that might allow the PTA to obtain or demonstrate advanced skills and knowledge? How might additional education or degrees assist the PTA in following a different career path beyond that of providing direct patient care? For those PTAs who later choose to become PTs, do their PT educational requirements differ from those of students who are not PTAs?

Where do you see yourself 5 years from now? Ten years from now? For those still in the early stages of their PTA education or careers, obtaining credentials and finally being able to work with patients is the culmination of years of hard work, and thinking about other career paths or additional formal education may seem uninteresting or unnecessary. However, although it is very important to celebrate the culmination of your entry-level education, it is just as important to review those steps you must take to begin your clinical career. It is never too early to consider the various options that are open to PTAs beyond that of providing direct patient care services and the ways to continue to develop a unique skill set. No matter where a PTA is in her educational journey, there are always "next steps" to consider in adding to her body of knowledge.

Lifelong Learning

Lifelong learning is defined by the APTA as "the systematic maintenance and improvement of knowledge, skills, and abilities through one's professional career or working life. Lifelong learning is the ongoing process by which the quality and relevance of professional services are maintained."[1] Being a lifelong learner and continuing to develop skills and knowledge are both necessary traits for success in the clinical setting and an expectation of the APTA, which states that PTAs "are obligated to engage in lifelong learning and are responsible for meeting and exceeding contemporary performance standards within their scope of work."[1] In addition, one of the eight Standards of Ethical Conduct for the Physical Therapist Assistant (see Chapter 5) specifically mandates this as part of the PTA's obligations.[2] It is an essential part of all PTAs' responsibility to their patients that they stay informed and continue to enhance their knowledge base and hands-on skills.

FOR REFLECTION

- Go back to Chapter 5 and find the specific standard within the Standards of Ethical Conduct that addresses lifelong learning. One of the standard's subcategories discusses changes in the profession. As physical therapy continues to evolve, how will you keep up to date with those changes?

For many PTAs, lifelong learning will mean more than what is required of every clinician. For some, it might mean seeking out formal recognition of additional acquired competencies or returning to school for additional education that will enhance their ability to work in different capacities while still working as a PTA. Still others might decide to take course work that builds on their PTA knowledge base but leads them to another role, such as someone who returns to school to become a PT. Many of those reading this chapter may have already demonstrated their ability to be lifelong learners by choosing to become PTAs after having worked in other careers or obtaining other degrees prior to beginning a PTA program. This chapter focuses on additional avenues of lifelong learning that can occur after the formal PTA education has concluded to help all future or current PTAs recognize that obtaining a PTA degree is not an end point, but a beginning!

The First Task: Passing the Licensure Examination

The first step in demonstrating lifelong learning occurs immediately after graduation for the vast majority of PTAs as they prepare for the Federation of State Boards of Physical Therapy (FSBPT) licensure examination. Preparing for the examination, although similar to preparing for any comprehensive examination that an individual PTA program may require, differs in that each educational program will have a slightly different emphasis from another in its curriculum and may use various testing formats. The licensure examination is a computerized test made up of 200 multiple-choice questions split into four sections of 50 questions each, with 1 hour allowed to complete each section. The questions are all free-standing, that is, no scenario in one question is connected to that of another. Only 150 questions of the 200 are actually scored; the other 50 are questions that are being tested for reliability and validity prior to being used as a scored question in an examination. There is no way of determining which questions are the "real" ones; therefore, all questions should be answered (there is no penalty for answering any of the 50 "trial" questions incorrectly). The raw score needed to pass varies from year to year, based on the determined difficulty of that year's examination. Raw scores are converted into scaled scores based on that year's level of difficulty, and a scaled score of 600 is required to pass.[3]

The content on the licensure examination (Table 14-1) may emphasize an area of content that did not receive as much emphasis in a student's academic curriculum, so when preparing for the examination students should consider using textbooks and other information from a variety of sources, not just notes and books from a single academic program. Various books and courses are designed specifically for preparing a soon-to-be graduate for the licensure examination. Most of these contain practice examinations (some are computerized) so that a student can become familiar with the style of testing and receive some feedback on content areas in which the student might need additional review. Although the time (and the expense) involved in taking a licensure examination preparation course may be daunting, it can be an extremely valuable investment and a way of demonstrating a commitment to being as successful as possible, right from the start. Complete information on the procedures required for obtaining initial licensure in a particular state should be obtained from that state's regulating board and the FSBPT.

Some states may have other requirements for initial licensure or renewal, for example requiring initial testing or periodic retesting of the laws specific to a state, known as a **jurisprudence examination.** The FSBPT is also investigating other mechanisms and tools for physical therapy practitioners to demonstrate continuing competence for licensure renewal, such as portfolios or competency examinations related to practice expertise areas.[4]

Finding Your First Position as a Physical Therapist Assistant

Many students will begin their job search even before they have graduated. In years past, this often consisted of reviewing the newspaper for help wanted ads. Today, employers commonly list open positions on their websites. This can make the job search more challenging for students and new graduates, not only because it requires going to each individual site to look for open positions, but also because many of these employers require applicants to submit their information electronically. Although this may sound like an easier way of navigating the job search, the requirements for standardized formats of applications and résumés, along with the volume of applications that are submitted, can make it challenging for one's application to stand out. Ensuring correct spelling and punctuation on any form submitted is a given. Just as important, the PTA's résumé needs to reflect the strengths and unique clinical background of that person. Considering that PTAs are generally applying for positions along with others who have similar education and clinical background, and that PTAs have a similar entry-level skill set, it is key that

Table 14-1   2013 National Physical Therapy Examination (NPTE) Test Content Outline—Physical Therapist Assistant[3]

Content Area Description (Number of Items)	Number of Items (acceptable range)	Items (%)
Physical Therapy Data Collection Cardiovascular/Pulmonary & Lymphatic Systems (6–7) Musculoskeletal System (12–13) Neuromuscular & Nervous Systems (8–10) Other Systems* (2–3)	**31 (28–33)**	**20.7**
Conditions/Diseases That Impact Effective Treatment Cardiovascular/Pulmonary & Lymphatic Systems (7–8) Musculoskeletal System (10–11) Neuromuscular & Nervous Systems (10–11) Other Systems* (12–18)	**42 (39–48)**	**28.0**
Interventions Cardiovascular/Pulmonary & Lymphatic Systems (10–11) Musculoskeletal System (15–17) Neuromuscular & Nervous Systems (13–14) Other Systems* (5–9)	**46 (43–51)**	**30.7**
Non-Systems Domains **Equipment & Devices; Therapeutic Modalities** Equipment & Devices (9–11) Therapeutic Modalities (11–13) **Safety & Protection; Professional Responsibilities; Research** Safety & Protection (3–4) Professional Responsibilities (2–3) Research & Evidence-Based Practice (2–3)	**31 (27–34)**	**20.7**
Total	150	100

* Other Systems include one or more of the following: Integumentary, Metabolic & Endocrine, Gastrointestinal, Genitourinary, and Systems Interactions.

Note: This represents only the 2013 content distribution; percentages may vary from year to year. (Reprinted with permission of the FSBPT.)

one's résumé highlights unique opportunities she may have had to develop improved self-confidence, enhanced time management, improved critical-thinking and problem-solving abilities, and stronger leadership skills, instead of a listing of the interventions delivered and the types of patient diagnoses with which one worked. Most academic institutions have career centers that can help students put together their résumés and the cover letters that usually accompany each individual job application.

The contacts that students make during their clinical experiences (or via APTA involvement and networking) are invaluable in job searches. Most students will use one or more CIs as references on their first job applications. In addition, many positions are first advertised via word of mouth, and clinical/APTA contacts often may pass on information to students about open positions at their sites or other locations. Some students will have the chance to interview, either for a real position or just for practice, at one or more of their clinical locations. This is an excellent opportunity to get feedback on one's résumé and interviewing skills. Doing some background research on the organization at which one is applying is highly recommended prior to an interview, as it prepares one to be able to ask more informed questions that focus on the organization and how it functions (rather than more generic questions concerning the position's benefits or work hours). The APTA has produced an online document that provides students and new graduates with questions to consider asking about an organization's business practices to be able to make informed decisions about whether a position at that site will be a good fit for them.[5]

In some states, once employed, students may be able to obtain temporary licenses that allow them to work as a PTA prior to taking the licensure examination, usually under more stringent supervision than required for a PTA who has obtained a permanent license.

FOR REFLECTION

- What strengths and skills would make your job application stand out from those of other new graduates?

Beyond Patient Care: Other PTA Roles in the Clinical Setting

Although direct patient care will probably always be the primary role for the PTA, there are other roles in which they can function, either along with or in lieu of performing direct patient care. Some of these additional aspects of a staff PTA's role are identified in the preceding chapter, which describes ways in which PTAs can develop and demonstrate leadership. This chapter highlights roles that the PTA might take after gaining additional experience or education.

FOR REFLECTION

- During your clinical experiences, what types of roles have you seen PTAs performing outside of direct patient care? Based on what you've read throughout this book, how did the role of the PTA compare with your expectations?

Clinical Instructor (CI)

For many PTAs, one of the first ways that they can demonstrate an interest in career development (as well as demonstrating leadership and professionalism) is by supervising a student who performs a clinical experience at the facility where the PTA works. Unlike some other health-care professions (i.e., nursing) that rely on paid faculty from the academic institution to supervise students in the clinic, the primary model used for clinical education in physical therapy relies on facility-employed clinicians who are willing to give back to the profession by volunteering to supervise a student, just as other clinicians once supervised them. Being a **clinical instructor (CI)** is a voluntary position but may be an expectation for everyone in the department. Clinicians usually are expected to have worked for at least a year before supervising a student,[6] but beyond that there is no specific requirement for being a CI other than an interest in working with students. Serving in this role is one of the most satisfying ways to give back to the profession, but what else is in it for the CI? Many CIs enjoy supervising a student because it gives them another way to keep up with changes in clinical practice through the student's academic curriculum. They see the opportunity to work with a student as a way in which each can enhance the other's education, the student with her up-to-date classroom knowledge and the CI with her clinical expertise. CIs traditionally do not get paid additional salary for supervising a student. However, some academic institutions may offer their CIs perks such as discounts on educational opportunities or access to the school's library system.

If a PTA serves as a CI, she should not be doing so in isolation, but rather as part of a PT/PTA team. Not only does being paired with a PT give the CI the opportunity for modeling the preferred PT/PTA relationship, but supervision provided by a PT CI (versus a PTA CI) may also be a requirement of certain third-party payers or state practice acts. Working with a PT as a CI team again requires strong communication and planning between the two to best plan the student's experience; as the PTA CI becomes more experienced, the PT CI may turn over primary responsibility for supervising the student to the PTA (again, within the constraints of payment sources and state laws), allowing the PTA CI to develop additional leadership skills.

How does a clinician know whether she is ready to be a CI? The APTA has some online self-assessments to use to determine readiness or need for additional preparation.[6] Another way of preparing is to attend a course through the APTA-sponsored Clinical Instructor Education and Credentialing Program. These courses were developed by the APTA "to develop and refine each participant's ability to teach, instruct, and guide the development of his or her students."[7] There is a basic as well as an advanced-level course; the basic course is designed for those who work with PT or PTA students, and the advanced course is specifically related to working with PT students. Many participants take the course prior to supervising their first student (some sites require the course for their CIs, and some academic programs likewise may require CIs to be credentialed, although this is not currently the norm). Other participants find that having had a student or two prior to taking the course helps give the course's content more relevance. One of the course's key concepts is that the planning, instructing, and assessing that PTs and PTAs do in their day-to-day activities naturally help them prepare for the process of supervising a student. The course's emphasis on this clinically obtained preparation, along with other information on learning styles, providing feedback, and working with the academic institution, helps many clinicians feel more confident in their ability to provide quality clinical education experiences.[8]

Supervision of Physical Therapy Aides

In some states, PTAs are legally allowed to participate in the supervision of a physical therapy aide or other support staff. The FSBPT's Model Practice Act discourages this practice, given that it is the PT's responsibility to direct and supervise all support personnel.[9] In some states, however, aides are allowed to perform tasks that assist a PTA in delivering interventions.[10] As allowed by law and best practice, working with a PT aide may be another way that a PTA can develop responsibility, leadership, and mentoring skills.

FOR REFLECTION

- Find out whether your state allows PTAs to participate in the supervision of physical therapy aides. If so, what are the legal parameters for providing that supervision?

Management and Ownership

In some situations, PTAs may serve in the role of a department manager or department liaison. Sometimes this occurs in part because the PTA is at a facility full-time, whereas the supervising PT floats between two or more different facilities, and it is logical to make the PTA the contact person for others when issues arise. In other cases, a PTA (usually with some type of additional advanced degree) may be chosen to serve as a departmental manager based on her expertise in business, finances, or management. This is somewhat controversial, given the nature of how PTAs must work under the direction and supervision of a PT, and by some it is interpreted as being out of line with current APTA Standards of Practice.[11] When an arrangement such as this is developed, it must be clear that the PTA is responsible for administrative duties, such as ensuring compliance with departmental and facility regulations, billing, risk management (see Chapter 10), program development, staffing, and scheduling. The ultimate responsibility for individual patient care decisions and the plan of care must continue to remain with the PT.[12]

Along with having opportunities for management, PTAs may have the opportunity to be involved with the ownership of a given clinic. Again, this is unusual and, in some minds, controversial, as it might imply that a PT as a staff person would be taking direction from a PTA owner. It is probably unusual to find a PTA who has an ownership interest in a clinic without a PT also being involved at a similar level, and the APTA has multiple positions that reiterate how the PT's autonomy in practice must be maintained regardless of employment relationships or business arrangements.[1,11,13]

Academia and the PTA

Some PTAs, after having gained some clinical experience, return to the place where their careers first started—the academic institution. According to the APTA's Normative Model of Physical Therapist Assistant Education, PTAs who have obtained a bachelor's degree and have 3 years of clinical experience meet the essential requirements for being an instructor for a PTA program. Other desired attributes may be a focused area of expertise, previous teaching experience, and some background in educational and instructional theory and methodology. To serve as the director of a PTA program, a PTA would be required to hold a master's degree.[14]

PTAs who do not have a bachelor's degree can still teach in a PTA program. Depending on the academic institution and its requirements for faculty rank, a PTA without a bachelor's degree may still be eligible to serve as an instructor in a PTA program or may hold a teaching position sometimes called "faculty assistant" or "laboratory assistant." Although this is usually not a role with full responsibility for managing a given course, faculty assistants may lead laboratory activities, assist with testing, or teach specified units of a course. When PTA faculty assistants work in courses with faculty members who are PTs, it gives students the opportunity to see the PT/PTA preferred relationship modeled even before they begin their clinical experiences.

PTAs are not just limited to teaching in PTA programs. For instance, St. Catherine University employs PTAs as faculty assistants in both its doctor of physical therapy (DPT) and PTA programs. When serving as faculty assistants in a DPT program, PTAs carry out many of the same responsibilities as in a PTA program, within the appropriate scope of work (for example, a faculty assistant who is a PTA would not participate in practical testing that assesses students' ability to perform a given examination procedure). The PT/PTA team is again modeled, this time for DPT students. These students gain valuable experience as they develop firsthand awareness of the education and knowledge base of the PTA, and they report that exposure to PTAs in the classroom environment has given them a greater understanding of how they should be supervised and used in the clinical setting.

Lifelong Learning Opportunities

The APTA has a position that expresses its expectation that PTAs are involved in lifelong learning. However, the APTA is not the only regulating body that holds an expectation that PTAs will further their knowledge base after graduation. Many states that regulate PTAs have some type of **continuing education (CE)** requirement for licensure (or their particular regulating level, if not licensure) renewal. Often this is spelled out in a practice act as a number of required contact hours (actual time spent in a CE activity, not counting breaks) or CE units (CEUs) per year (or other time period); one CEU is in most cases equated to 10 contact hours.

CE has been broadly defined as "participation in educational opportunities reflecting a commitment to lifelong learning."[14] The types of courses and other educational opportunities that qualify for CE credit vary from state to state. The various types of CE offerings are usually categorized within the total CE requirement, with a certain number of CEUs necessary in some categories and only a limited number of CEUs credited toward the total requirement in other categories. In addition, to receive full credit for them, many CE activities need to have been preapproved for credit by that state's regulating body for physical therapy. The CE requirements for PTAs vary considerably from state to state, and they may or may not be the same number of hours as required for PTs.[10] Usually, a course brochure will indicate whether it has been approved for CE credit; always contact the state board if there are questions regarding whether a given course or activity will qualify.

Types of CE opportunities include courses and conferences sponsored by the state APTA chapter, local colleges and universities, and health-care organizations. CE courses are also run by private companies and may be held in different locations across the country. These could be as short as an hour or two, a series of weekly courses, or a full-day or weekend seminar. The APTA also provides CE courses in all of these formats; in addition, it provides many home study courses (these consist of readings followed by examinations that must be returned to the APTA for credit), along with webinars and other online course work available through the APTA website. Finally, the national association sponsors two annual conferences with multiple days of CE opportunities for PTs and PTAs on a huge range of topics sponsored by the organization as a whole or by various APTA sections. The APTA's Combined Sections Meeting is held every winter and is solely devoted to CE; the Annual Conference and Exposition of the American Physical Therapy Association, held every summer, is usually preceded by the House of Delegates meeting and other governance-related activities. The APTA has a policy that every annual conference is expected to include meetings and programming specifically for the PTA.[15]

FOR REFLECTION
■ Find out the CE requirements (if any) for your state.

Continuing Your Formal Education

The APTA's House of Delegates passed a position in 2006 that an associate degree was the minimal degree required for PTAs,[16] and this currently continues to be the degree awarded after completion of entry-level PTA programs. Many PTA graduates, however, either enter PTA programs with other degrees or obtain one (or more) after completing a PTA program. The academic majors a PTA might pursue are endless. Business, education, and leadership degrees, at either a bachelor's or master's level, are frequently used to enhance the PTA's role in the clinical setting. This section highlights some unique opportunities available for PTAs who choose to continue their formal education.

Degree Completion Options

A few years ago, it was not uncommon for PTAs to consider returning to school for a bachelor's degree, only to find that because of the specialized nature of their PTA academic curriculum they would not receive any transfer credit for most of their previous education. To prevent PTAs from having to start over completely if they choose to return to school, a number of PTA programs now have developed bachelor's **degree completion programs** as subsequent educational options for their graduates. These programs allow graduates to apply the credits earned in their PTA program course work toward credits required for a bachelor's degree. Because most PTA programs are housed in institutions that offer only 2-year associate's degrees, they usually must partner with another school that offers baccalaureate degrees to provide this opportunity. However, a few PTA programs are housed in 4-year institutions and thus are able to offer degree completion options within their own institution. These programs may or may not be exclusively designed for PTAs (graduates of other 2-year health-care programs, such as occupational therapy assistants, may also be eligible), but they most often have some type of health-care focus and result in the student receiving a degree in a major such as health-care management.[17] A list of degree completion programs that accept previous PTA courses for credit is posted on the APTA website.[18]

Many educators and PTAs believe that as the role of the physical therapist and the demands of the current clinical environment have grown, the associate degree does not allow enough time to best prepare entry-level PTAs to be the support personnel of choice in today's physical therapy clinic. In 2012, the House of Delegates requested a study to be performed to determine the feasibility of moving the entry-level PTA degree to a bachelor's degree instead of an associate degree. The results of this study, although identifying some barriers and concerns with changing the degree level, recognized many advantages to additional education for the PTA. However, it did not reach a clear conclusion as to whether that additional education should occur as part an expanded entry-level degree instead of during post-entry-level education.[19] Currently, the Commission on Accreditation for Physical Therapy Education (CAPTE) is able to accredit only associate degree PTA programs, and until such time as it is able to accredit entry-level baccalaureate programs, the standard for the entry-level degree level is unlikely to change. As degree completion programs do not require CAPTE accreditation, there has been a growing interest in degree completion programs specific to the role of the physical therapist assistant that further develop the skills and knowledge obtained via the entry-level degree and subsequent clinical experience. There is currently one degree completion program in which graduates receive a bachelor of science as a physical therapist assistant,[20] and other programs that are in the process of developing similar degree completion options.

PTA to PT

Currently, there are only two academic programs identified by CAPTE as offering a special cohort program designed specifically for PTAs who wish to become PTs.[21] In the past, when the PT degree was at a bachelor's level, a few more of these types of programs existed. However, the conversion to an advanced entry-level degree requirement for PTs has made the transition from PTA to PT more challenging; it requires the PTA to have additional prerequisites and, usually, a bachelor's degree before beginning a PT program. If the PTA entry-level degree ever transitions to an entry-level bachelor's degree, it is possible that there will be new PTA-to-PT programs that develop as a result. In the meantime, the course work of some degree completion programs currently may include classes that fulfill the prerequisite requirements for a DPT program.

If a PTA does decide to return to school to become a PT, she is generally given very little, if any, credit for her PTA education or experience (except in specialized PTA-to-PT programs such as the ones described here) and does not get an exemption for any DPT program course work. However, the PTA's previous education and clinical experience certainly give her unique insight into the PT's role and PT/PTA interaction, as well as a comfort level with patient care delivery and documentation that most likely will be greater than that of her classmates.

FOR REFLECTION

- Do you think a PTA who subsequently becomes a PT should get credit for previous course work or experience? Why or why not? If this is difficult to answer, review Chapter 1, which discusses similarities and differences between PTA and PT programs.

Obtaining a Related Degree

Some PTAs choose to return to school to make themselves more marketable in the physical therapy workforce. Others do so because they have found that they want to use their health-care background in a related but different field, such as occupational therapy or nursing. It is possible that a PTA who subsequently wants to obtain training in another health-care field might be able to receive curriculum credit for some of her previous liberal arts or PTA program course work, depending on the new field that she is entering and its specific requirements. Those who are interested in obtaining an additional degree in a health-care or exercise-related field are encouraged to contact the specific program directly to ask about receiving credit for previous education or work experience.

A handful of PTA programs offer transition programs for other health-care practitioners who are interested in advancing their career options by becoming a PTA. Some PTA programs have begun to offer their curriculum in a specialized manner to cohorts of students who enter the program with a specific background, such as athletic training, massage therapy, or military training as a physical therapy technician. Students who are in one of these programs may receive PTA program course credit for specific areas of work experience, allowing them to complete their PTA degree with fewer courses. Any PTA program offered in this manner needs to have CAPTE approval for its modified curriculum prior to admitting students. Because this type of program is occurring in physical therapy, it is possible that it might also occur at some point in other fields in which a group of PTAs could be the specialized cohort.

Lifelong Learning Through Involvement in Research

Keeping up with current evidence and research in the physical therapy profession is critical to the provision of quality care, and the mechanisms for reviewing such research are discussed in Chapter 13. PTAs need not be limited to just reviewing current evidence; they can also participate in its development. In reality, however, most PTAs, unless they are in academia, have limited opportunity to participate in original clinical research studies such as randomized controlled trials (RCTs) or to share those results in a written, peer-reviewed article. There is no reason why a PTA could not be involved in this type of work, but there are other ways in which PTAs, even as students, are more likely to perform research and present their results. One of the first ways that students are often asked to educate others is by developing and presenting an **in-service,** a brief (usually shorter than 1 hour) presentation to members of the physical therapy or rehabilitation department in which a clinical experience is being performed. These presentations are usually on a topic with particular relevance to that clinical site, chosen either by the student or her CI, and could include (but are not limited to) subject areas such as:

- An update on a diagnosis seen or procedure commonly used in the clinic
- A review of current evidence related to an intervention of interest
- Information about PTA utilization and/or the PT-PTA relationship, if PTs at that clinical site are less familiar with the role of the PTA
- A legislative or regulatory update, such as proposed changes in a state statute, APTA position, or issues related to health-care reform

After the person providing the in-service presents the information on the chosen topic, those attending are generally given the opportunity to ask questions of the presenter. In-service activities can be as formal as desired, but often are presented in the style of a meeting, with everyone gathered at a table, rather than with the presenter standing or at a podium. Because of the busy nature of the clinical environment, in-service activities are frequently conducted during lunch, with participants eating while learning.

Another format for sharing information that students may have an opportunity to experience is a **case study.** A case study is a report of one particular patient's "story," in which the reviewer presents the patient's history, describes the interventions the patient received, and then discusses the outcomes related to those interventions. In Chapter 13, case studies are identified as being low on the hierarchy of levels of evidence.[22] However, this does not mean that they are without value. Case studies are often performed when the patient presents with unusual symptoms, a rare diagnosis, or a unique combination of diagnoses or impairments that do not fit the mold of those that are traditionally represented in higher-level evidence such as RCTs. They may also be conducted to highlight a new intervention technique or a patient whose response to intervention was surprising or complicated, stimulating additional research on the topic. Although evidence in a case study rarely can be generalized to an entire population, it can provide insight into how others might proceed if faced with a similarly challenging situation.[23]

Case studies can be presented in written format, just like other types of research, but they are frequently reported using the **poster presentation** format. Posters can be used to highlight any type of research, not just case studies. In fact, the two previously mentioned national APTA conferences traditionally feature hundreds of poster presentations on all types of research formats. A poster presentation's content is similar to that featured in an article abstract (see Chapter 13); it summarizes the highlights of each section of the research methodology as it was performed, along with the results that were obtained. Especially at the national level, poster sizes are often prescribed and are limited to relatively small dimensions, requiring the poster developer to be very concise and clear in the material presented.[24]

Another format for presenting results of research is called a **platform presentation.** Platform presentations are those in which researchers review the findings of an original study in a short time frame (often fewer than 20 minutes). PowerPoint slides or other types of visual aids are used to supplement the speaker's commentary.[24] Again, because of the limited time available, the material presented must be concise, but the platform presentation allows for oral commentary that might be challenging to summarize in the written format of a poster.

Achieving and Demonstrating Advanced Skill Development Through the APTA

As discussed in Chapter 9, in response to PTAs' complaints that there was no mechanism for them to demonstrate advanced competency, in 2005 the APTA began its **Recognition of Advanced Proficiency for the Physical Therapist Assistant.** Being honored in such a way by the APTA has given these PTAs formal recognition of their expertise in a particular area of physical therapy beyond that of the entry-level clinician. Other benefits for the recipient, as described by the APTA, include gaining increased confidence in one's abilities, potential career advancement opportunities, and reinforcement of the value of lifelong learning.[25] However, to provide more structure and consistency in the expertise required to demonstrate advanced proficiency, the mentoring and education that was required to obtain this designation has now become a component of the APTA's **Advanced Proficiency Pathways (APPs).** As of 2016, PTAs can apply to participate in one of six APPs that address the following content areas:

- Acute Care
- Cardiopulmonary
- Geriatrics
- Oncology
- Pediatrics
- Wound Management

The APPs include course work common to all of the proficiency areas, other courses unique to that APP, and formal mentoring from a PT selected by the PTA. Participation in an APP provides additional structure and timelines for accomplishing advanced proficiency requirements in a more uniform way between participants.[26]

The APTA as a Means of Career Development

The first step in accessing all of the various resources the APTA has to offer is by becoming a member. The rationale for PTAs being members of the APTA is addressed in detail in Chapter 9 and includes much more than just what a PTA can receive from doing so. However, an undeniably significant benefit of membership is that of having better access to the numerous lifelong learning and career development opportunities available through the APTA. Although many of the APTA's conferences and CE offerings on the state and national levels are available to nonmembers, being a member usually allows the PTA to participate in these at a significantly lower cost. In addition, membership in the APTA will keep PTAs better informed of changes within the profession and about available career advancement opportunities. Many states participate in the APTA's Career Starter Dues program that offers discount membership rates to **new professionals,** those PTs or PTAs who have graduated in the past 5 years. The APTA has a dedicated page on its website for new professionals, with links to information to the Career Center, where job opportunities are posted, along with information about student loan repayment, licensure, career development, and networking.[27]

One of the most common ways of networking with others in the APTA is by joining a **section,** a subgroup of members with a common interest in a particular area of practice or diagnosis, such as pediatrics or oncology. Each section may have multiple **special interest groups (SIGs),** which have an even more concentrated focus on a particular subset of practice.[28] Many state chapters also have SIGs; it isn't necessary to be part of the national section/SIG to participate in the SIG at the state level.

APTA Sections and Associated Special Interest Groups[28]

Academy of Acute Care Physical Therapy
- Total Joint Replacement

Academy of Geriatric Physical Therapy
- Balance & Falls
- Bone Health
- Cognitive and Mental Health
- Health Promotion and Wellness
- Residency/Fellowship

Academy on Clinical Electrophysiology & Wound Management
- Wound Management

Aquatics

Cardiovascular & Pulmonary

Education
- Academic Faculty
- Clinical Education
- PTA Educators

(box continues on page 274)

APTA Sections and Associated Special Interest Groups (continued)

Federal Physical Therapy
Hand Rehabilitation
Health Policy & Administration
- Global Health
- Technology

Home Health
Neurology
- Balance & Falls
- Brain Injury
- Degenerative Diseases
- Spinal Cord Injury
- Stroke
- Vestibular Rehabilitation

Oncology
- HIV/AIDS
- Hospice and Palliative Care
- Lymphedema
- Pediatric Oncology

Orthopaedic
- Animal Rehabilitation
- Foot and Ankle
- Imaging
- Occupational Health Physical Therapy
- Pain Management
- Performing Arts

Pediatrics
- Academic and Clinical Educators
- Adolescents & Adults with Developmental Disabilities
- Early Intervention
- Hospital-based Physical Therapy
- Neonatology
- Pediatric Sports-Fitness
- School-based Physical Therapy

Private Practice
- Administrators Council
- Industry Partner
- National Student SIG

Research
- Biomechanics Research
- Early Career Researchers
- Evidence Based Practice
- Qualitative Research

APTA Sections and Associated Special Interest Groups (continued)

Sports Physical Therapy
- Emergency Response
- Female Athlete
- Golf and Golf Performance
- Hip
- Knee
- Pediatric Sports Fitness
- Physically Challenged Athlete
- Professional/Collegiate Therapist
- Shoulder
- Sports Performance Enhancement

Women's Health

Lifelong learning through the APTA can occur in ways other than CE opportunities. Chapter 9 describes some of the organized participation opportunities available to PTAs within the APTA. But how does a PTA initiate being involved at that level? For many PTAs, it might begin with attending a meeting for PTAs at the state level. Many of the state chapters have a SIG specifically for PTAs and their issues.[28] Attending a PTA SIG meeting is a great way to keep up with the issues that affect PTAs, to network with other PTAs in the same state, and to keep the role of the PTA visible to the chapter's membership. Because the national average of PTAs who are members is small (hovering around 7 percent in recent years)[29] and an even smaller number of those are active in their PTA SIGs, new members are always welcomed.

Many PTAs, it has been noted, join other SIGs or committees within their state chapter. Depending on the chapter's bylaws, PTAs may have an opportunity to serve in leadership positions on a chapter committee or on their chapter's board of directors. The vast majority of states report having PTAs in these roles.[30] In addition, some state licensing boards also have specially designated PTA positions for which any PTA can apply, but the person chosen to serve is often appointed (by a governor or other state official).[9]

Those PTAs looking for an even greater level of involvement in the APTA might consider serving as a state representative to the PTA Caucus. The PTA Caucus is the representative group for PTAs within the APTA's current governance structure. PTA Caucus representatives have a number of responsibilities:

- Representing the views of the PTAs within their states and sharing them with others in the national organization
- Serving as a communication liaison between individual members and the PTA Caucus as a whole
- Sharing the viewpoints of PTAs with their state's PT membership at large and with their House of Delegates representatives

In some states, PTA Caucus representatives are elected; in others they are appointed (and some states report difficulty in filling their PTA Caucus representative positions). Terms are usually for 2 years, and many states provide at least partial funding for the PTA Caucus representative to attend the two in-person PTA Caucus meetings that are held each year (one at the Combined Sections Meeting and another before the annual meeting of the House of Delegates). Within the PTA Caucus, there are additional opportunities for participation and leadership development by running for an elected office (one of four Delegate positions, Chief Delegate, Alternate Delegate, or one of three Nominating Committee positions, all 2-year terms).[31]

Another route of service for PTAs on a national level is to be a member of an appointed volunteer group. These opportunities generally fall into three categories:[32]

- Committees that assist the Board of Directors with ongoing APTA work;
- Work groups developed to assist APTA staff with association management; and
- Task forces that focus on a specific emerging issue for a short time and then disband.

PTAs can indicate their interest in participating in one of these by submitting their name and background information to the Volunteer Interest Pool page on the APTA website. The APTA Board of Directors then fills vacancies on these groups from that applicant pool, as appropriate for the needs and qualifications required in each group.[32]

Experienced PTAs with an interest in the education process can serve the profession by becoming an item writer for the FSBPT PTA licensure examination or by becoming a site reviewer for CAPTE's accreditation process. To write questions for the licensure examination, PTAs must be licensed and have 2 years of clinical experience, but they do not need to have experience writing test questions. After attending a 3-day training session in which they prepare an initial 10 questions, item writers are expected to develop at least 30 more questions over a 3-month period. They are given a small stipend (currently $150) for every 20 questions that are submitted and approved for the test item bank.[33]

PTAs must also have experience to serve as on-site reviewers for accreditation and reaccreditation of PTA educational programs. There are spots on every site review team for a PTA serving as an educator or clinician (along with a PT and a non-PT basic scientist, health-care educator, or administrator). PTAs must have 2 years of experience in the clinical or academic setting, depending on which role they fill on the team. In addition, on-site reviewers must be APTA members and remain so during the time spent serving in that role (a term of service is 5 years, with the option of serving multiple terms). Training workshops are held regularly for new reviewers, with additional training required of those serving as review team leaders.[34]

SUMMARY

The end of formal education in a PTA program merely ends the first phase of the PTA's educational journey. Whether by continuing to learn through one's first position as a PTA, subsequent acquired work experience and continuing education, completing additional academic degrees, or participating in research activities, the PTA fulfills the mandate of the APTA that "PTAs are responsible for meeting and exceeding contemporary performance standards within their scope of work."[1] PTAs have opportunities, through membership and involvement in the APTA, to demonstrate achievement of advanced skill and knowledge and to advocate for the role of the PTA through involvement in state chapter activities, national-level advisory panels, the PTA Caucus, and other national PT-related organizations. Taking advantage of the limitless possibilities for lifelong learning and career advancement that are available is a duty that all PTAs owe to their patients, but the additional personal rewards of doing so can result in an extremely fulfilling lifetime career!

REFERENCES

1. American Physical Therapy Association. Professional development, lifelong learning and continuing competence in physical therapy (HOD P05-07-14-14). http://www.apta.org/uploadedFiles/APTAorg/About_Us/Policies/Professional _Development/ProfessionalDevelopmentLifelongLearning.pdf. Updated 2012. Accessed September 5, 2015.
2. American Physical Therapy Association. Standards of ethical conduct for the physical therapist assistant. http://www.apta.org/uploadedFiles/APTAorg/About _Us/Policies/Ethics/StandardsEthicalConductPTA.pdf. Updated 2015. Accessed August 13, 2015.
3. Federation of State Boards of Physical Therapy. NPTE Candidate Handbook. http://www.fsbpt.org/FreeResources/NPTECandidateHandbook.aspx. Updated 2015. Accessed August 14, 2015.
4. Federation of State Boards of Physical Therapy. Continuing competence. https://www.fsbpt.org/Licensees/ContinuingCompetence.aspx. Updated 2015. Accessed September 5, 2015.
5. American Physical Therapy Association. Considerations for practice opportunities and professional development. http://www.apta.org/CareerManagement/ConsiderationsforOpportunities/. Updated 2010. Accessed September 7, 2015.
6. American Physical Therapy Association. Clinical educator development. http://www.apta.org/Educators/Clinical/EducatorDevelopment/. Updated 2014. Accessed September 5, 2015.
7. American Physical Therapy Association. Credentialed clinical instructor program. http://www.apta.org/CCIP/. Updated 2015. Accessed August 14, 2015.
8. Buccieri KM, Schultze K, Dungey J, et al. Self-reported characteristics of physical therapy clinical instructors: a comparison to the American Physical Therapy Association guidelines and self-assessments for clinical education. *J Phys Ther Educ*. 2006;20(1):47-55.
9. Federation of State Boards of Physical Therapy. The model practice act for physical therapy: a tool for public protection and legislative change. 5th ed. https://www.fsbpt.org/Portals/0/documents/free-resources/MPA_5thEdition2011 .pdf. Updated 2011. Accessed August 13, 2015.
10. Federation of State Boards of Physical Therapy. Licensure reference guide. https://www.fsbpt.org/FreeResources/RegulatoryResources/LicensureReferenceGuide. Updated 2011. Accessed August 13, 2015.
11. American Physical Therapy Association. Standards of practice for physical therapy (HOD S06-13-22-15). http://www.apta.org/uploadedFiles/APTAorg/

About_Us/Policies/Practice/StandardsPractice.pdf. Updated 2013. Accessed August 20, 2015.

12. American Physical Therapy Association. Principles of professionalism guiding physical therapist business relationships (BOD P10-09-04-09). http://www.apta.org/uploadedFiles/APTAorg/About_Us/Policies/Practice/PrinciplesProfessionalismBusinessRelationships.pdf. Updated 2012. Accessed September 5, 2015.

13. American Physical Therapy Association. Autonomous physical therapy practice (HOD P06-06-18-12). http://www.apta.org/uploadedFiles/APTAorg/About_Us/Policies/Practice/AutonomousPTPractice.pdf. Updated 2012. Accessed September 5, 2015.

14. American Physical Therapy Association. *A Normative Model of Physical Therapist Assistant Education: Version 2007.* Alexandria, VA: American Physical Therapy Association; 2007.

15. American Physical Therapy Association. Programs for physical therapist assistant members (HOD Y06-76-25-65). http://www.apta.org/uploadedFiles/APTAorg/About_Us/Policies/Meetings/ProgramsPTAMembers.pdf. Updated 2012. Accessed September 5, 2015.

16. American Physical Therapy Association. Educational degree requirements for physical therapist assistants (HOD P06-03-25-22). http://www.apta.org/uploadedFiles/APTAorg/About_Us/Policies/Education/EducationalDegreeQualificationsPTA.pdf. Updated 2012. Accessed September 5, 2015.

17. St. Catherine University. Healthcare management. https://www2.stkate.edu/healthcare-mgmt-ewo/home. Updated 2015. Accessed September 5, 2015.

18. American Physical Therapy Association. Career resources for PTAs. http://www.apta.org/PTA/Careers/. Updated 2014. Accessed September 7, 2015.

19. American Physical Therapy Association. RC 20-12 feasibility study for transitioning to an entry-level baccalaureate physical therapist assistant degree. *2014 House of Delegates Handbook.* 2014:240-241.

20. Pima Medical Institute. Bachelor of science in physical therapist assistant program. http://pmi.edu/Programs/Bachelors/Bachelor-of-Science-Physical-Therapist-Assistant. Updated 2015. Accessed September 7, 2015.

21. Commission on Accreditation in Physical Therapy Education. Education programs bridging from PTA to PT. http://www.capteonline.org/Programs/Bridge/. Updated 2014. Accessed September 6, 2015.

22. Straus SE, Glasziou P, Richardson WS, Haynes RB. *Evidence-Based Medicine: How to Practice and Teach It.* 4th ed. Philadelphia, PA: Elsevier Churchill Livingstone; 2011.

23. Portney LG, Watkins MP. *Foundations of Clinical Research: Applications to Practice.* 3rd ed. Upper Saddle River, NJ: Prentice-Hall; 2009.

24. Carter R, Lubinsky J, Domholdt E. *Rehabilitation Research: Principles and Applications.* 4th ed. St. Louis, MO: Elsevier Saunders; 2011.

25. American Physical Therapy Association. PTA recognition of advanced proficiency. http://www.apta.org/PTARecognition/. Updated 2016. Accessed January 22, 2016.

26. About the PTA Advanced Proficiency Pathways (APP) program. http://www.apta.org/APP. Updated 2015. Accessed January 22, 2016.

27. American Physical Therapy Association. Information for new professionals. http://www.apta.org/NewProfessionals/. Updated 2015. Accessed September 7, 2015.

28. American Physical Therapy Association. Special interest groups (SIGs). http://www.apta.org/apta/components/public/sigs.aspx?navID=10737421974. Updated 2015. Accessed September 5, 2015.

29. American Physical Therapy Association. 2013 PT/PTA market share by state. Membership Development Statistics Web site. http://www.apta.org/MembershipDevelopment/Statistics/. Updated 2013. Accessed September 7, 2015.

30. American Physical Therapy Association. 2015 House of Delegates background papers. The Hub: File Library: Background Papers Web site. http://communities.apta.org/p/do/sd/sid=1215&type=0. Updated 2015. Accessed September 7, 2015.

31. American Physical Therapy Association. PTA caucus. http://www.apta.org/PTA/Caucus/. Updated 2015. Accessed September 5, 2015.

32. American Physical Therapy Association. APTA volunteer groups. http://www.apta.org/VolunteerGroups/. Updated 2015. Accessed September 6, 2015.

33. Federation of State Boards of Physical Therapy. Item writer flyer. http://www.fsbpt.org/Portals/0/documents/volunteers/ItemWriterFlyer20110325.pdf. Updated 2011. Accessed September 6, 2015.

34. Commission on Accreditation in Physical Therapy Education. CAPTE accreditation handbook. http://www.capteonline.org/AccreditationHandbook/. Updated 2015. Accessed 2015, September 6.

Name _____

REVIEW

1. What is a jurisprudence examination? Does your state require new graduate PTAs to take a jurisprudence exam?

_____

_____

_____

2. What are the advantages to the clinician for serving as a CI?

_____

_____

_____

_____

3. Other than writing an article, what are two other ways that a PTA might be involved in discussing or presenting research?

_____

_____

_____

_____

(questions continue on page 282)

Application

1. Review the list of proficiency categories within the APTA's PTA Advanced Proficiency Pathways (APPs). Identify one that you might be interested in pursuing, and explain why you chose that one.

_____

_____

_____

_____

2. Think about where you see your career leading you, and identify goals for the next 5 years to help measure your success in achieving your plan. What type of lifelong learning or career development will you need to pursue to reach your goals? Fill in the accompanying chart to help you plan your path toward your goals.

Goal	Time Frame for Achieving Goal	Learning Opportunities (CE, Networking, Mentoring, Volunteering) That Might Help in Goal Achievement

Index

Note: Page numbers followed by "b," "f," and "t" indicate boxes, figures, and tables, respectively.